The Effective Management of Osteoporosis

The Effective Management of Osteoporosis

Edited by

David H Barlow MA BSc MD FRCOG FMedSci
Nuffield Professor of Obstetrics and Gynaecology,
University of Oxford, Oxford, UK

Roger M Francis MB ChB FRCP
Reader in Medicine (Geriatrics), University of Newcastle-upon-Tyne & Honorary
Consultant Physician, Musculoskeletal Unit, Freeman Hospital,
Newcastle-upon-Tyne, UK

Andrew Miles MSc MPhil PhD
Professor of Public Health Policy and Health Services Research
& UK Key Advances Series Organiser,
University of East London, UK

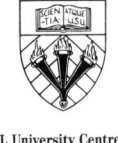

UeL University Centre for
Public Health Policy &
Health Services Research

AESCULAPIUS MEDICAL PRESS
LONDON SAN FRANCISCO SYDNEY

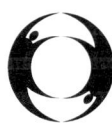

National
Osteoporosis
Society

Published by

Aesculapius Medical Press (London, San Francisco, Sydney)
Centre for Public Health Policy and Health Services Research
Faculty of Science and Health
University of East London
33 Shore Road, London E9 7TA, UK

British Library Cataloguing in Publication Data
A catalogue record for this book is available from the British Library

ISBN 1 903044 08 1

While the advice and information in this book are believed to be true and accurate at the
time of going to press, neither the authors nor the publishers nor the sponsoring institutions
can accept any legal responsibility or liability for any errors or omissions that may be made.
In particular (but without limiting the generality of the preceding disclaimer) every effort
has been made to check drug usages; however, it is possible that errors have been missed.
Furthermore, dosage schedules are constantly being revised and new side-effects recognised.
For these reasons, the reader is strongly urged to consult the drug companies' printed
instructions before administering any of the drugs recommended in this book.

Further copies of this volume are available from:

Claudio Melchiorri
Research Dissemination Fellow
Centre for Public Health Policy and Health Services Research
Faculty of Science and Health
University of East London
33 Shore Road, London E9 7TA, UK

Fax: 020 8525 8661
email: claudio@keyadvances4.demon.co.uk

Typeset, printed and bound in Britain
Peter Powell Origination & Print Limited

Contents

Contributors

David H Barlow MA BSc MD FRCOG FMedSci, Nuffield Professor of Obstetrics and Gynaecology, University of Oxford, Oxford

Glen M Blake PhD, Department of Nuclear Medicine, Guy's Hospital, London

Cyrus Cooper DM FRCP MRC, Environmental Epidemiology Unit, University of Southampton, Southampton

Elaine Dennison MSc MRCP, Environmental Epidemiology Unit, University of Southampton, Southampton

Ignac Fogelman MD, Department of Nuclear Medicine, Guy's Hospital, London

Roger M Francis MB ChB FRCP, University of Newcastle-upon-Tyne and Musculoskeletal Unit, Freeman Hospital, Newcastle-upon-Tyne

Allan L Harris LRCP MRCS, Haxby Group Practice, Haxby and Wiggington Health Centre, Wigginton, York

Cynthia P Iglesias MSc Department of Health Studies and Centre for Health Economics, University of York, York

Gordana M Prelevic MD DSc FRCP, Department of Medicine, Royal Free & University College Medical School, London

Harpal Randeva MRCP, Sir Quinton Hazell Molecular Medicine Research Centre, Department of Biological Sciences, University of Warwick, Warwick

David M Reid MD FRCP, Department of Health Studies and Centre for Health Economics, University of York, York

Janice Rymer MD MRCOG FRANZCOG, Consultant and Senior Lecturer, Department of Obstetrics and Gynaecology, St Thomas' Hospital, London

Michael D Stone BA DM FRCP, Bone Research Unit, University of Wales College of Medicine, Llandough Hospital, Penarth

Anne M Sutcliffe BSc RGN DN HV, Musculoskeletal Unit, Freeman Hospital Newcastle-upon-Tyne

Jonathan H Tobias MB BS MA MD PhD FRCP, Rheumatology Unit, Bristol Royal Infirmary, Bristol

David J Torgerson PhD, Department of Health Studies and Centre for Health Economics, University of York, York

Jane Turton MB MSc MRCGP, Bone Research Unit, University of Wales College of Medicine, Llandough Hospital, Penarth

Preface

There has been a dramatic increase in our understanding of the pathogenesis, impact and management of osteoporosis over the past 25 years. Osteoporosis was previously regarded as an inevitable consequence of ageing aggravated by the menopause in women. Hormone replacement therapy (HRT), calcium and vitamin D supplements were occasionally used in the treatment of osteoporosis, but there was little evidence of their effectivness at that time.

We are now aware that osteoporosis also affects men and younger women. We also know that the seeds of osteoporosis are sown early in life, as genetic factors, dietary calcium intake and exercise during childhood all determine peak bone mass at maturity and may therefore influence the subsequent risk of osteoporotic fractures. It is now clear that bone loss with advancing age is due not only to the menopause in women, but also to factors such as reduced physical activity, vitamin D insufficiency and secondary hyperparathyroidism. There are also a number of underlying conditions which accelerate the development of osteoporosis, including amenorrhoea, hypogonadism in men, oral corticosteroid therapy and organ transplantation, all of which may cause severe osteoporosis and fractures.

The major osteoporotic fractures are those of the forearm, spine and hip. It has been estimated that one in three women and one in twelve men in the UK will experience one of these three fractures during their lifetime. These fractures are associated with excess mortality, substantial morbidity and vast health and social service expenditure.

Fortunately, the past decade has seen the development of accurate methods of measuring bone density. These bone density measurements can be used to diagnose osteoporosis before fractures occur and to assess the future risk of fracture. We also now have a number of treatments, which have been shown to increase bone density and decrease the risk of fractures. These include HRT, selective oestrogen receptor modulators, bisphosphonates and calcium and vitamin D supplements.

The progress in understanding about the causes, impact and treatment of osteoporosis was recognised by the publication by the Department of Health of their Advisory Group on Osteoporosis Report in 1994. This advised health authorities to purchase services for osteoporosis patients, including bone density measurements for specified clinical indications. The Report also suggested that the Royal College of Physicians developed Guidelines for osteoporosis management. Comprehensive evidence-based guidelines for the management of osteoporosis were subsequently published by the Royal College of Physicians in 1999.

A national symposium was held with the National Osteoporosis Society at the Royal College of Physicians of London in November 1999, which highlighted the key advances in the effective management of osteoporosis. This volume provides a useful review of the major presentations at this meeting, but also includes new information that has been published since then.

Doctors and health professionals are increasingly overwhelmed by clinical information, so we have aimed to provide an up-to-date fully referenced text which is as succinct as possible but as comprehensive as necessary. Consultants and their trainees interested in osteoporosis will find it of particular use as part of their continuing professional development and specialist training. We anticipate that the book will also prove useful to clinical nurse specialists as a reference text and to commissioners of health services as the basis for discussion and negotiation of health contracts with their practising colleagues.

In conclusion, we thank Organon Laboratories Ltd. for the grant of educational sponsorship which helped to support the national symposium at the Royal College of Physicians of London, at which synopses of the constituent chapters of this book were presented.

David H Barlow MA BSc MD FRCOG FMedSci
Roger M Francis MB ChB FRCP
Andrew Miles MSc MPhil PhD

PART 1

Identification of osteoporosis

Chapter 1

Epidemiology of osteoporotic fractures

Elaine Dennison and Cyrus Cooper

Introduction

Osteoporosis is a skeletal disorder characterised by low bone mass and micro-architectural deterioration of bone tissue with a consequent increase in bone fragility and susceptibility to fracture (Consensus Development Conference 1991). It is a widespread condition, often unrecognised in clinical practice, which may have devastating health consequences through its association with fragility fractures. The term 'osteoporosis' was first used in the nineteenth century as a histologic description for aged bone tissue, but its clinical consequences were not appreciated until Sir Astley Cooper recognised that hip fractures might result from an age-related reduction in bone mass or quality over 150 years ago. Since one disadvantage of a fracture-based definition is that diagnosis and treatment will be delayed when prevention is considered optimal treatment, an expert panel convened by the World Health Organisation (WHO) has suggested that both low bone mineral density (BMD) and fracture be combined in a stratified definition of osteoporosis (World Health Organisation 1994).

   Population based data from the United States suggest that while the majority of white women aged under 50 years have normal bone density, osteoporosis becomes increasingly prevalent with advancing age (Melton 1995). However, prospective studies indicate that the risk of osteoporotic fracture increases continuously as BMD declines with a 1.5–3-fold increase risk of fracture for each standard deviation fall in BMD (Cummings *et al.* 1993). There does not appear to be a threshold value for BMD above which the fracture risk is stable, and the risk gradient for this relationship is as steep as that between blood pressure and stroke. Use of this density-based definition allows early diagnosis and therefore early initiation of preventive strategies.

The size of the problem

Using the WHO criteria, it has been estimated that most American women under the age of 50 years have normal BMD and that osteoporosis is rare. With advancing age, an increasing number of women have osteoporosis, so that by the age of 80 years 27 per cent are osteopenic and 70 per cent are osteoporotic at the hip, lumbar spine or forearm. Epidemiological studies from North America (Melton 1995) have estimated the lifetime risk of common fragility fractures to be 17.5 per cent for hip fracture, 15.6 per cent for clinically diagnosed vertebral fracture and 16 per cent for distal forearm fracture among white women aged 50 years. Corresponding risks among men are 6 per cent, 5 per cent and 2.5 per cent . Estimates from Europe suggest that around 23 per cent of women aged 50 years and over have osteoporosis according to the WHO definition. Fracture rates in Britain are somewhat lower than in the United States: for women lifetime fracture incidence rates are 14 per cent, 11 per cent and 13 per cent at hip, spine and distal forearm respectively, while for men the corresponding figures are 3 per cent, 2 per cent and 2 per cent (Dennison & Cooper 1996) (Table 1.1).

Table 1.1 Impact of osteoporotic fractures in British men and women. (Reproduced with permission from Dennison *et al.* 1996)

		Hip	*Vertebra*	*Wrist*
Lifetime risk (%)				
	Women 50 y	14	11	13
	Men 50 y	3	2	2
Mean age (years)		79	67	65
Mortality (relative survival)		0.83	0.82	1.00
Functional impairment (%)		30	10	10

Epidemiology of fractures

Although osteoporotic fractures are more common among women than men, the ratio describing incidence in the two sexes is not the same for all fracture types, and varies considerably with age (Cooper & Melton 1992a) (Figure 1.1). In young people, fractures of the long bones predominate, often following substantial trauma, and the incidence is greater in young men than in young women. Above the age of 35 years, overall fracture incidence in women climbs steeply, so that rates in women become twice those of men. At least 1.3 million fractures in the United States each year have been attributed to osteoporosis, assuming that 70 per cent of all fractures in persons aged 45 years or over are due to the condition (Iskrant & Smith 1969). Most fractures in the elderly are due to minor or moderate trauma. They usually occur in falls from the standing position, but have been known to occur spontaneously, and occur more frequently in the winter months in temperate countries. The majority occur during falls indoors, rather than as a result of slipping on icy surfaces. One explanation that has been suggested to account for this observation is the possibility of impaired neuromuscular function at lower temperatures. Alternatively, bone density may suffer adversely from reduced vitamin D production in winter as a result of reduced sunlight exposure. The sex difference is more pronounced in white populations, with oriental and black populations tending towards similar age-adjusted rates in men and women (Melton 1991). The three sites most closely associated with osteoporosis are the hip, spine and distal forearm. The epidemiological characteristics of these three types of fracture differ, suggesting the influence of different factors, including the varying relative contribution of bone strength and trauma to fracture risk at each site.

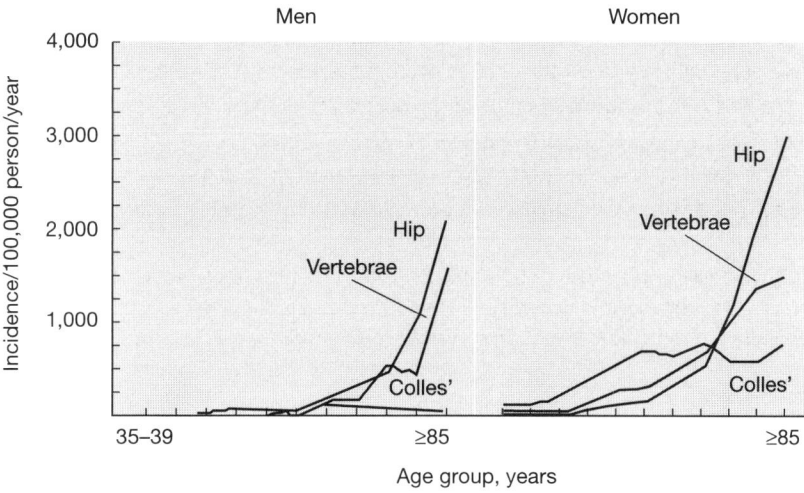

Figure 1.1 Age-specific incidence rates for hip, vertebral and distal forearm fractures in men and women. (Reproduced with permission from Cooper *et al.* 1992)

Hip fracture

This represents the most serious complication of osteoporosis and is associated with considerable morbidity and mortality (Cooper *et al.* 1993) (Figure 1.2). Its incidence increases exponentially with age in both men and women. However, at all ages beyond 50 years, the incidence in women is about twice that in men, and since there are more elderly women than men, about 80 per cent of all hip fractures occur in women. Worldwide, there were an estimated 1.66 million hip fractures in 1990; about 1,197,000 in women and 463,000 in men (Cooper *et al.* 1992).

The vast majority of hip fractures follow a fall from standing height or less. The likelihood of falling rises with age and is greater in women than men; a survey in Oxford, England reported that about one in three women aged 80–84 years had had a fall in the previous year, and this rose to nearly half of women aged 85 years and over (Winner *et al.* 1989). Only about 1 per cent of all falls lead to a hip fracture however, because the amount of trauma delivered to the proximal femur depends upon the orientation of the fall (Gibson 1987).

Although hip fractures occur 15 years later, on average, than spine and wrist fractures, they are associated not only with a greater risk of functional impairment and institutionalisation, but also with a 20 per cent mortality rate within the first year (Baudoin *et al.*1996). Most deaths observed with hip fracture occur soon after the fracture. Excess mortality is particularly marked in men over 75, and this may reflect comorbidity, dementia and a range of attributes related to secondary osteoporosis (Poor *et al.* 1995). Quality of life in survivors may also be severely impaired; one

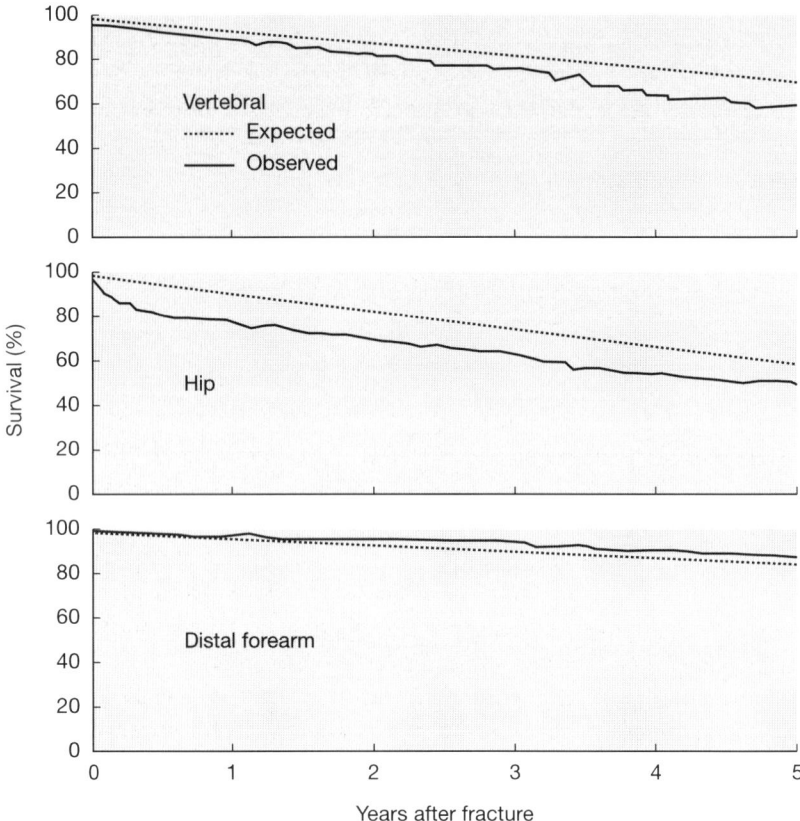

Figure 1.2 Five-year survival after the diagnosis of fracture. (Reproduced with permission from Cooper *et al.* 1993)

year post fracture, 40 per cent of patients are unable to walk independently, 60 per cent are unable to do at least one activity of daily living, and at least 80 per cent are unable to do at least one independent activity of daily living, such as shopping or driving (Cooper 1997).

Incidence rates in hip fracture vary substantially from one population to another. Hip fracture is far less common among non-whites than whites, and there is also substantial variation within populations of a given race and gender. Age-adjusted hip fracture incidence rates are higher among Scandinavian residents than comparable populations.

In North America, and even within Europe, hip fracture rates vary over sevenfold from one country to another (Johnell *et al.* 1992). This marked variation in hip fracture incidence suggests an important role for environmental factors, and highlights a need for additional studies.

Vertebral fracture

Vertebral fractures show a more linear pattern of increasing incidence with age among women than men, and are associated with excess mortality, possibly through coexisting frailty. It has been noted that among patients with clinically diagnosed vertebral deformity in Rochester, Minnesota, USA, observed mortality was greater than predicted over a five year period among both men and women (Cooper *et al.* 1993). This is consistent with the observation that low bone density per se predicts earlier death (Browner *et al.* 1991).

Accurate epidemiological data on vertebral fracture have been difficult to collect for two reasons: first, there is no universally recognised definition of vertebral deformity from lateral thoracolumbar x-rays, and secondly, the majority of vertebral fractures are asymptomatic. The application of recently developed definitions to various population samples in the USA has permitted estimation of the incidence of new vertebral deformities in the general population (Melton *et al.* 1993). The incidence of new vertebral deformity has been estimated to be about three times that of hip fracture for post-menopausal white women (Cooper & Melton 1992b). The age-adjusted female:male ratio for these deformities is 1.9, with only about one third recognised clinically. The most frequently affected levels are T8, T12 and L1, corresponding with the weakest regions in the spine. Trauma plays a far larger role in the aetiology of vertebral deformities in men, especially in younger patients.

Large epidemiological studies have also recently been conducted throughout Europe: in the European Vertebral Osteoporosis Study, 15,570 men and women aged 50–79 years were selected from population registers in 36 European centres (O'Neill *et al.* 1996). Lateral spine radiographs were taken according to a standardised protocol and evaluated centrally. The overall prevalence of morphometrically defined vertebral deformity was 12 per cent in men and women. The prevalence increased with age in both sexes (Figure 1.3), although the gradient was steeper among women than among men. There was substantial geographic variation, with the highest rates observed in Scandinavian countries (O'Neill *et al.* 1996). The risk of vertebral deformity among men was significantly elevated in those with very high levels of physical activity (Silman *et al.* 1997), suggesting the aetiological significance of trauma. Risk was elevated among women with a late menarche or early menopause (O'Neill *et al.*1997). In this, as in other studies, number of vertebral deformities was associated with height loss and history of back pain in the year prior to the interview (Cooper *et al.* 1995).

Previous vertebral deformities have been shown to increase the risk of subsequent vertebral deformities by seven- to tenfold (Ross *et al.* 1991). In a population-based retrospective cohort study in Rochester, Minnesota, residents aged less than 70 years of age who were radiologically diagnosed with one or more vertebral deformities were followed up for the development of subsequent limb fractures. The standardised morbidity ratios of observed to expected fractures were 1.7 (95 per cent CI 1.3–2.2)

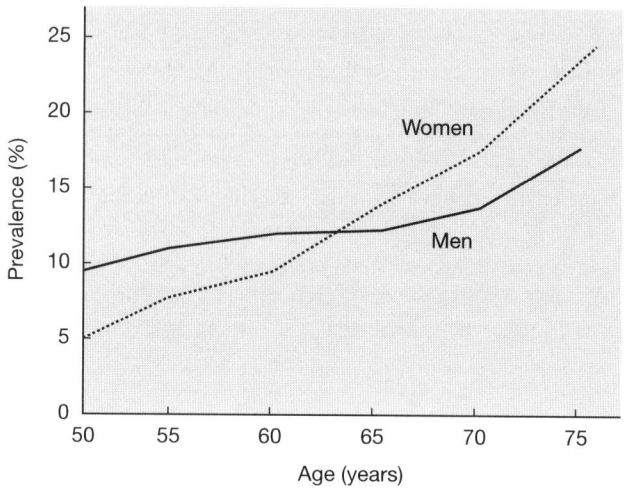

Figure 1.3 Prevalence of vertebral deformity in European men and women with advancing age (European Vertebral Osteoporosis Study). (Reproduced with permission from O'Neill TW *et al.* 1996)

for the hip, 1.4 (95 per cent CI 1.0–1.8) for the forearm and 1.5 (95 per cent CI 1.3–1.8) for any limb fracture. This increased risk was apparent among men and women, and was more marked in subjects with vertebral deformities associated with moderate or minimal trauma than with severe trauma.

The Study of Osteoporotic Fractures, a prospective study of 9,704 US women aged 65 years or older, has also studied the relationship between prevalent vertebral deformity and incident osteoporotic fracture (Black *et al.* 1999). Prevalent vertebral deformity (assessed morphometrically) was associated with a fivefold increased risk of sustaining a further vertebral deformity; the risk of hip fracture was increased 2.8 fold (95 per cent CI 2.3–3.4) and the risk of any non-vertebral fracture 1.9 fold (95 per cent CI 1.7–2.1), after adjustment for age and calcaneal BMD. Although there was a small increased risk of wrist fracture, this was not significant after adjustment for age and BMD.

Wrist fracture

The epidemiology of wrist fracture seems distinct from that of hip and vertebral fracture. Distal forearm (Colles) fracture almost always results as a consequence of a fall onto an outstretched hand. These fractures show a steep rise in incidence during the perimenopausal period among women, but a plateau thereafter. In men there is no apparent increase in incidence of wrist fracture with age. In white women, the incidence increases linearly between the ages of 40 and 65 and then stabilises, while in men the incidence remains constant between 20 and 80 years (Cooper & Melton

1992a). A much stronger sex ratio exists for this fracture than for most others and this has been estimated to be 4:1 in favour of women. Although geographic variation exists, a partial explanation may be methodological considerations of case ascertainment, since less than 20 per cent of forearm fracture patients are hospitalised. A winter peak is again demonstrated, but this is probably due to falls outside on icy surfaces. The plateau with age in women may be due to mode of falls; later in life a woman is more likely to fall onto a hip than an outstretched hand as her neuromuscular co-ordination deteriorates.

The Rochester Minnesota project has also been used to ascertain the ability of distal forearm fractures to predict future fractures (Cuddihy *et al.* 1999). Among residents who experienced their first distal forearm fracture aged 35 years or older, and excluding fractures that occurred on the same day as the index forearm fracture, hip fracture risk was increased 1.4-fold in women (95 per cent CI 1.1–1.8) and 2.7-fold in men (95 per cent CI 0.98–5.8). Excess risk in women was confined to those individuals who sustained their first forearm fracture at age 70 years or greater. By contrast, vertebral fracture was increased at all ages, with a 5.2-fold (95 per cent CI 4.5–5.9) increase in risk among women and a 10.7-fold (95 per cent CI 6.7–16.3) increased risk among men.

Other fractures

Fractures at several other sites, including the proximal humerus, pelvis and proximal tibia, exhibit the features of osteoporotic fractures. There is an excess of these fractures in women, incidence rates increase with advancing age and most result from only mild or moderate trauma. Furthermore, these fractures are associated with low appendicular bone mass with a similar magnitude to hip and vertebral fractures (Seeley *et al.* 1991).

Economic costs

The financial costs of osteoporotic fracture are difficult to estimate accurately because they not only include hospital admission and long-term residential care, but also more indirect costs such as loss of working days and pharmacological preventive strategies. Although it is primarily hip fracture that is associated with hospitalisation and failure to return home, there are considerable costs associated with outpatient visits, nursing care and days off work for all fracture types. Reported medical costs for initial stabilisation of a hip fracture range from US$1,900 in Portugal to US$9,000 in Greece. In the United Kingdom (population 60 million), the annual cost to the healthcare system from osteoporotic fractures has been estimated at £942 million (Torgerson & Cooper 1998).

Future projections

Life expectancy is increasing worldwide, and it is estimated that the number of individuals aged 65 years and over will increase from the current figure of 323 million to 1,555 million by the year 2050 (Cooper & Melton 1992a). These demographic changes alone can be expected to cause the number of hip fractures occurring worldwide to increase from 1.66 million in 1990 to 6.26 million in 2050. While about half of all hip fractures among elderly people in 1990 took place in Europe and North America, by 2050 the rapid aging of the Asian and Latin American populations will result in the European and North American contribution falling to only 25 per cent. In addition, although age-adjusted rates appear to have levelled off in the northern part of the United States (Jacobsen *et al.* 1991) and in the United Kingdom (Spector *et al.* 1990) (Figure 1.4), rates continue to increase in Hong Kong (Lau *et al.* 1990). On the basis of current trends, hip fracture rates might increase in the United Kingdom from · 46,000 in 1985 to 117,000 in 2016 (Hoffenberg *et al.* 1989).

There are three broad explanations for these trends. The first might reflect the influence of some increasingly prevalent risk factor for osteoporosis such as decreased physical activity, more frequent falls or increased rates of oophorectomy (Melton *et al.* 1987). An alternative explanation might be increasing frailty in the elderly. The explanation for the reversal of the trend is less clear because no specific population-based strategies have been employed but the increasing availability of medical care may be important. Alternatively, the initial increase in incidence could represent a cohort effect adversely influencing bone mass or the risk of falling. Generational effects explain some of the secular trends in adult height during this century, leading to an increase in hip axis length which may increase the risk of hip fracture.

Incidence rates for fractures at other skeletal sites have also risen during the last half century. Studies from Malmo, Sweden (Obrant *et al.* 1989), have suggested age-specific secular increases for distal forearm, ankle, proximal humerus, and vertebral fractures. These changes in vertebral fracture rate are particularly important as they point to an increasing prevalence of osteoporosis, rather than falling, as an explanation for these trends.

Table 1.2 shows the projections for the number of hip fractures throughout Europe in 2000, 2020 and 2050, assuming constant incidence rates over that period. Demographic changes alone will account for an almost threefold increase in the number of hip fractures among men and women by the year 2050; even a 1 per cent annual increase in the age-adjusted incidence of hip fracture would produce almost doubling of these rates by the year 2050.

Conclusion

Large epidemiological studies have now provided good evidence regarding risk factors for osteoporosis, at a time when potent therapeutic agents to retard bone loss and prevent fractures have been developed. A coherent strategy is now required, not only to treat patients with established osteoporosis, but also to develop public health strategies relating to bone mass and falling. Without such measures, the financial and health-related costs of osteoporosis look set to rise exponentially in future generations.

Table 1.2 European projections for hip fracture

Year	No. of hip fractures (x 10³)	
	Male	Female
2000	88	326
2020	139	456
2050	230	742

Source: European Community 1998

References

Baudoin C, Fardellone P, Bean K, Ostertaq-Ezembe A, Hervy F (1996). Clinical outcomes and mortality after hip fracture: a 2 year follow-up study. *Bone* **18**, S149–157.

Black DM, Arden NK, Palermo L, Pearson J, Cummings SR (1999). Prevalent vertebral deformities predict hip fractures and new vertebral deformities but not wrist fractures. *J Bone Miner Res* **14**, 821–28.

Browner WS, Seeley DG, Vogt TM, Cummings SR (1991). Non-trauma mortality in elderly women with low bone mineral density. *Lancet* **338**, 355–358.

Consensus Development Conference (1991). Prophylaxis and treatment of osteoporosis. *Osteoporosis Int* **1**, 114–17.

Cooper C (1997). The crippling consequences of fractures and their impact on quality of life. *Am J Med* 12S–19S.

Cooper C & Melton LJ III (1992a). Epidemiology of osteoporosis. *TEM* **3**, 224–229.

Cooper C & Melton LJ III (1992b). Vertebral fracture: how large is the silent epidemic? *BMJ* **304**, 793–794.

Cooper C, Atkinson EJ, Jacobsen SJ, O'Fallon WM, Melton LJ III (1993). Population-based study of survival after osteoporotic fractures. *Am J Epidemiol* **137**, 1001–1007.

Cooper C, Campion G, Melton LJ III (1992). Hip fracture in the elderly: A world wide projection. *Osteoporosis Int* **2**, 285–289.

Cooper C, O'Neill TW, Egger P *et al.* (1995) Vertebral deformities: clinical impact and relation to fractures at other sites. *J Bone Miner Res* **10**, S145.

Cuddihy MT, Gabriel SE, Crowson CS, O'Fallon WM, Melton III LJ (1999). Forearm fractures as predictors of subsequent osteoporotic fractures. *Osteoporosis Int* **9**, 469–75.

Cummings SR, Black DM, Nevitt MC *et al.* (1993). Bone density at various sites for prediction of hip fractures. *Lancet* **341**, 72–75.

Dennison E & Cooper C. The Epidemiology of Osteoporosis. *British Journal of Clinical Practice* **50**, 33–36.

Gibson MJ (1987). The prevention of falls in later life. *Dan Med Bull* **34**, 1–24.

Hoffenberg R, James OFW, Brocklehurst JC *et al.* (1989). *Fractured Neck of Femur: Prevention and Management.* Summary and recommendations of a report of the Royal College of Physicians, London, pp 8–12.

Iskrant AP, Smith RW Jr (1969). Osteoporosis in women 45 years and over related to subsequent fractures. *Public Health Rep* **84**, 33–8

Jacobsen SJ, Goldberg J, Miles TP, Brody JA, Stiers A (1991). Seasonal variation in the incidence of hip fracture among white persons aged 65 years and older in the United States, 1984–7. *Am J Epidemiol* **133**, 996–1004.

Johnell O, Gullberg B, Allander E *et al.* (1992). The apparent incidence of hip fracture in Europe: a study of national register sources. *Osteoporosis Int* **2**, 298–302.

Lau EMC, Cooper C, Wickham C, Donnan S, Barker DJP (1990). Hip fracture in Hong Kong and Britain. *Int J Epidemiol* **19**, 1119–21

Melton LJ III (1991). Differing patterns of osteoporosis across the world. In *New Dimensions in Osteoporosis in the 1990s. Hong Kong* (Chesnut C ed.) Excerpta Medica, Asia, pp13–18.

Melton LJ III (1995). How many women have osteoporosis now? *J Bone Miner Res* **10**, 175–177.

Melton LJ, Chrischilles EA, Cooper C, Lane AW, Riggs BL (1992). How many women have osteoporosis? *J Bone Miner Res* **7**, 1005–1010.

Melton LJ III, Lane AW, Cooper C, Eastell R, O'Fallon WM, Riggs BL (1993). Prevalence and incidence of vertebral deformities. *Osteoporosis Int* **3**, 113–119.

Melton LJ III, O'Fallon WM, Riggs BL (1987). Secular trends in the incidence of hip fractures. *Calcif Tissue Int* **41**, 57–64.

Obrant KJ, Bengner U, Johnell O, Nillson BE, Sernbo I (1989). Increasing age-adjusted risk of fragility fractures: a sign of increasing osteoporosis in successive generations? *Calcif Tissue Int* **44**, 157–67.

O'Neill TW, Felsenberg D, Varlow J, Cooper C, Kanis JA, Silman AJ (1996). The prevalence of vertebral deformity in European men and women: the European Vertebral Osteoporosis Study. *J Bone Miner Res* **11**, 1010–1028

O'Neill TW, Silman AJ, Naves-Diaz M E et al. (1997).Influence of hormonal and reproductive factors on the risk of vertebral deformity in European women. *Osteoporosis Int* **7**, 72–8

Poor G, Atkinson EJ, O'Fallon WM, Melton LJ III (1995). Determinants of reduced survival following hip fractures in men. *Clin Orthop* **319**, 260–265.

Ross PD, Davis JW, Epstein R, Wasnich RD (1991). Pre-existing fractures and bone mass predict vertebral fracture incidence. *Ann Intern Med* **114**, 919–23.

Seeley DG, Browner WS, Nevitt MC *et al.* (1991). for the Study of Osteoporotic Fractures Research Group. Which fractures are associated with low appendicular bone mass in elderly women? *Ann Intern Med* **115**, 837–842.

Silman AJ, O'Neill TW, Cooper C *et al.* (1997). Influence of physical activity on vertebral deformity in males and females: results from the European Vertebral Osteoporosis Study. *J Bone Miner Res* **12**, 813–9.

Spector TD, Cooper C, Lewis AF (1990). Trends in admissions for hip fracture in England and Wales, 1968–1985. *BMJ* **300**, 1173–1174.

Torgerson D & Cooper C (1998). Osteoporosis as a candidate for disease management: Epidemiological and cost of illness considerations. *Disease Management and Health Outcomes* **3**, 207–214.

Winner SJ, Morgan CA, Evans JG (1989). Perimenopausal risk of falling and incidence of distal forearm fracture. *BMJ* **298**, 1486–8.

World Health Organization (1994). *Assessment of Fracture Risk and its Application to Screening for Postmenopausal Osteoporosis.* WHO technical report series, WHO, Geneva.

Chapter 2

The individual at risk of osteoporosis: advances in the use of techniques for the identification of high risk groups within the general population and identification of the individual with active disease

Glen M Blake and Ignac Fogelman

Introduction

The term 'osteoporosis' is frequently used without any clear indication of its meaning. Thus, osteoporosis may be used to describe both the clinical outcome (i.e., a low trauma fracture) and the changes in bone tissue that precede a fracture. A useful and inclusive definition is that proposed by the Consensus Development Conference (1993), namely *'A disease characterised by low bone mass and microarchitectual deterioration of bone tissue leading to enhanced bone fragility and a consequent increase in fracture risk'*. Osteoporosis has been called the silent epidemic since there are no associated symptoms or warning signs other than fracture, which is clearly too late. For this reason, the decision to initiate preventive treatment must be based on assessments of patients using factors that are indicative of a high risk of a future fracture. Of these, the two most useful are age and a low bone mineral density (BMD) (Hui *et al.* 1988; Black *et al.* 1992; Cummings *et al.* 1993). In addition, patients who have previously suffered a fragility fracture are at increased risk of further fractures independently of age and BMD (Melton *et al.* 1999).

Measurements of BMD are widely recognised as being very effective at identifying those patients who are at a higher than average risk of fracture (Marshall *et al.* 1996). However, they cannot be used to make specific predictions of particular individuals who will later actually sustain a fracture. This is because the occurrence of osteoporotic fractures is multifactorial, involving other factors such as chance accidents and a propensity to falls. Hence not all patients identified at high risk by BMD measurements will actually suffer fractures, while a proportion of individuals thought to be at lower risk will sustain a fracture.

Progress during the last decade in the identification and treatment of patients at high risk of an osteoporotic fracture has turned around four important developments:

- the introduction and subsequent widespread availability of new instrumentation for quickly and conveniently measuring BMD

- publication of the findings of several large epidemiological studies into the relationship between BMD and fracture risk
- the report by a World Health Organisation (WHO) task group which defined osteoporosis as a BMD value at the spine, hip or forearm 2.5 or more standard deviations (SD) below the mean for healthy young adults, with or without a history of previous fracture (World Health Organisation 1994)
- publication of the findings of several large clinical trials which show that some new treatments for osteoporosis can reduce fracture incidence by up to 50 per cent. We shall review each of these developments in turn.

Recent developments in bone densitometry

Since its introduction in 1987, dual X-ray absorptiometry (DXA) has become widely recognised as the 'gold standard' for the evaluation of BMD (Genant *et al.* 1996; Grampp *et al.* 1997; Blake *et al.* 1999). The advantages of DXA include the ability to measure BMD in the spine and hip, which are widely recognised as the fracture sites that entail the most serious consequences for the patient; short scan times (typically 30 seconds for a spine or hip scan using a fan-beam instrument); low radiation dose (equivalent to less than a day's exposure to natural background radiation for most instruments (Njeh *et al.* 1999); highly reproducible measurements. The precision of BMD measurements of the lumbar spine and the total femur region in the hip are both approximately 1per cent. Allied to the high precision is the excellent longterm stability of DXA equipment. Provided the manufacturers' instructions on regular instrumental quality control scans using phantoms are followed carefully, DXA can be used to monitor long-term changes in BMD at selected sites such as the lumbar spine (Eastell 1998).

BMD and fracture risk

The most important evidence that BMD measurements are a useful indication of future fracture risk comes from large prospective studies such as the Study of Osteoporotic Fractures (SOF), a study of over 9,000 women aged 65 years and over living in four cities in the United States (Black *et al.* 1992; Cummings *et al.* 1993). Such studies are analysed using a 'gradient of risk' model in which the fracture risk is assumed to increase exponentially as BMD decreases (this is a slight over simplification: in practice the logit function ($\text{logit}(p) = \log(p/1\text{-}p)$) is correlated with BMD instead of $\log(p)$ to ensure that the probability of fracture p does not exceed 1.0 at low BMD). The 'gradient of risk' is expressed by the odds ratio (OR) which is defined as the increased risk of fracture for a 1 population SD decrease in BMD. Results from several large studies show that values for the OR are typically about 2.0 (Marshall *et al.* 1996). It should be recognised that such statistical modelling is only an approximation in the same sense that linear regression analysis is frequently applied to scatter plots or distribution data are modelled with gaussian curves.

Nevertheless, an indication of the way the model often gives a good description of the findings of fracture studies is shown by another popular way of presenting such data, namely by dividing the baseline BMD values into four quartiles and plotting the fracture risk separately for each. Figure 2.1 shows data from the hip fracture study of Cummings *et al.* (1993) plotted in this way. In Cummings' study patients in the lowest quartile of hip BMD had an 8.5 times greater risk of hip fracture than subjects in the highest quartile.

The OR value is the most important figure of merit for assessing the predictive value of BMD measurements at any selected site in the skeleton. The larger the OR value, the better the measurements are able to discriminate those patients who will later suffer a fracture. Marshall *et al.* (1996) collated the findings of the prospective fracture studies in a meta-analysis. Figure 2.2 is a summary of their conclusions plotted to show the OR figures for BMD measurements at the spine, hip, forearm and calcaneus to predict osteoporotic fractures of the spine, hip, forearm or at any site in the skeleton. These data are generally recognised as showing that the best predictor of fracture risk at a given skeletal site is a BMD measurement at that site. Thus, Figure 2.2 shows that hip BMD is a better predictor of hip fracture (OR = 2.6) than spine fracture (OR = 1.8). Similarly, spine BMD is a better predictor of spine fracture (OR = 2.3) than hip fracture (OR = 1.6). That spine BMD performs somewhat less well than hip BMD may reflect the effects of degenerative disease in the spine

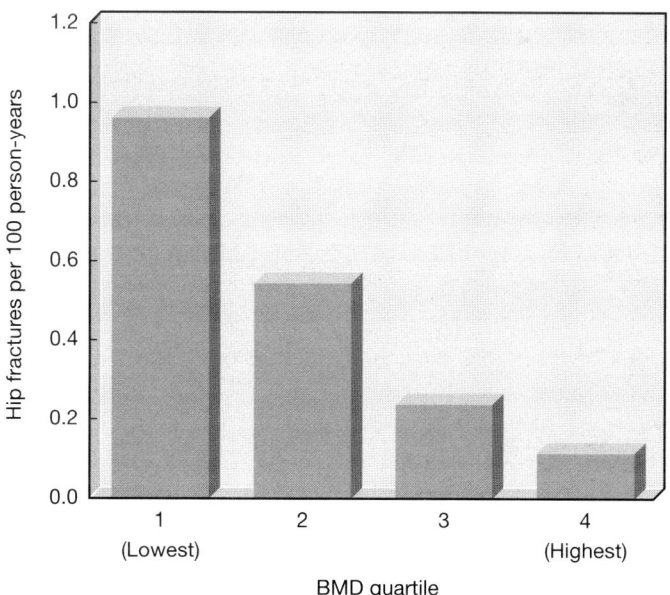

Figure 2.1 Incidence of hip fracture by BMD quartile for femoral neck bone density (data from Cummings *et al.* 1993)

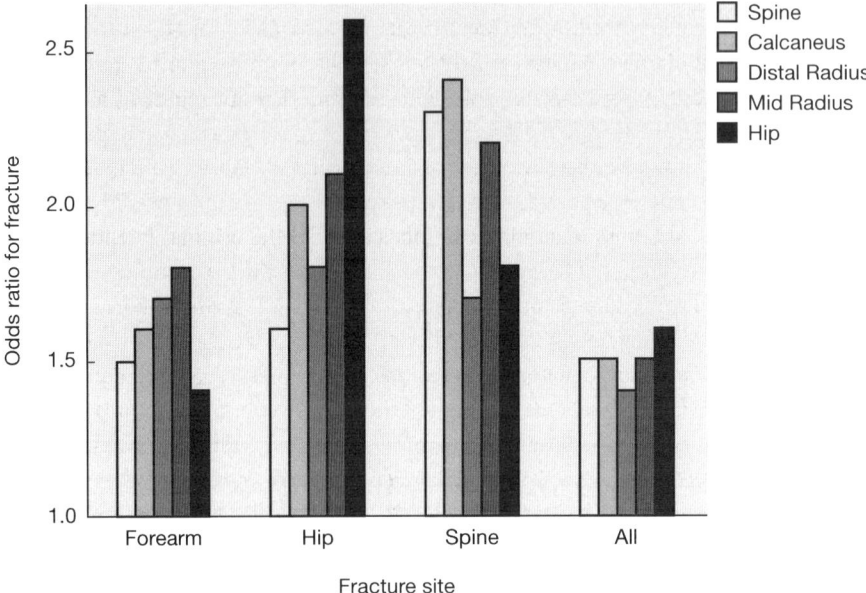

Figure 2.2 Odds ratios for fractures at different skeletal sites for bone density measurements in the spine, calcaneus, distal radius, mid-radius and hip (data from meta-analysis of prospective studies collated by Marshall *et al.* 1996)

which can adversely affect the quality of BMD measurements at this site in patients aged 65 and over. However, the data in Figure 2.2 should not be overinterpreted. It is clear that the statistical errors in the OR data remain relatively large for even the largest prospective studies and that the findings to date cannot be regarded as proving unequivocally that any one BMD measurement site is superior to any other. In particular, it is notable that when judged by the ability to predict *any* osteoporotic fracture, the different BMD sites appear equivalent. However, it may be necessary to qualify the above remarks for hip fractures, since in the SOF study hip BMD measurements were shown to be (marginally) statistically significantly better predictors of hip fracture than measurements at any other site in the skeleton (Cummings *et al.* 1993).

The World Health Organisation (WHO) task group report

The report by the WHO task group published in 1994 marked an important development, since, for the first time it allowed a consensus on how patients with osteoporosis should be recognised before they suffer a fracture rather than afterwards. The WHO report classified skeletal status using a patient's T-score value which expresses their BMD result in terms of the difference from the mean BMD for a young adult population divided by the young adult population SD. Based on the WHO criteria, patients with a T-score ≤ -2.5 are regarded as being at high risk of sustaining a low trauma fracture and are classified as having osteoporosis. Those who meet this criterion but have already suffered a low trauma fracture are said to have *established osteoporosis*. Those with a T-score between -2.5 and -1.0 are regarded as being at intermediate risk and are classified as having *osteopenia*, while those with a T-score ≥-1.0 are at low risk and regarded as normal. The WHO criteria have commanded a lot of attention because they provide clinicians with a rational basis on which to diagnose and treat patients, although it should be emphasised that the original intention was to provide a definition for epidemiological studies rather than a guide to treatment. The T-score threshold of -2.5 was chosen on the basis that about 30 per cent of post-menopausal women aged 50 years or over have a T-score ≤ -2.5 at the spine, hip or forearm and this figure equates approximately with their lifetime risk of fracture. Additionally, the threshold is sufficiently low that very few pre-menopausal women are included (< 1 per cent). Despite the simplistic rationale, the WHO definition of osteoporosis met an important need and has now acquired a predominant role in the clinical interpretation of BMD scans. In comparison, less attention has been paid to the WHO definition of osteopenia, probably because it captures too high a percentage of post-menopausal women, especially when multiple sites in the skeleton are assessed. Its use as a basis for treatment decisions might therefore prove prohibitively expensive.

New treatments for osteoporosis

Recent developments of new therapies for treating osteoporosis are having a major influence on requirements for bone densitometry services. While most experts consider hormone replacement therapy (HRT) to be the treatment of choice for osteoporosis, only a minority of women are prepared to take this treatment long-term. However, in recent years new treatments such as bisphosphonates and selective oestrogen receptor modulators (SERMs) have become available and are of proven efficiency. With the publication of the fracture intervention trial (FIT) it is apparent that bisphosphonates such as alendronate are capable of reducing the incidence of both spinal and femoral fractures by 50 per cent (Black *et al.* 1996). In addition, the importance of calcium and vitamin D supplementation, particularly in the elderly, has become recognised (Chapuy *et al.* 1992). SERMs such as raloxifene have the advantages of HRT with regard to protecting the skeleton and cardiovascular system, but without stimulating the endometrium or breast tissue (Delmas *et al.* 1997).

The availability of powerful new treatments for osteoporosis is expanding the need for bone densitometry services. Thus it is becoming more widely accepted that patients should have a spinal BMD measurement before commencing glucocorticoid therapy (Reid 1997). Various groups have published guidelines for the use of BMD measurements in at risk populations, but these are not yet widely applied in practice (Barlow 1994; Kanis *et al.* 1997). In many of these situations, for example women with an early menopause or those with previous thyrotoxicosis or primary hyperparathyroidism, results of a BMD scan can influence patient management.

The future of bone densitometry services

A number of developments are pointing the way to the future evolution of bone densitometry services, together with some significant revisions in the way scan results are interpreted. An important issue is the perception that conventional DXA scanning of the spine and hip is expensive because it requires patients to be referred to a hospital. Although there are now more than 200 DXA units installed in the United Kingdom, many of these are used for research studies so their availability for referrals from General Practitioners is limited. There is therefore great interest in the future role of peripheral skeletal measurements which could be carried out either in general practice or at small local hospitals. The measurement of forearm BMD is well established having been available for almost 30 years. A new generation of equipment has been developed in which the ^{125}I radionuclide source used in early forearm devices has been replaced by a low voltage X-ray generator thus making the widely recognised advantages of DXA available for forearm densitometry (Blake *et al.* 1999). A more radical development is the increasing interest in quantitative ultrasound (QUS) measurements of bone, which have the capability of providing a cheap, portable, radiation-free assessment of skeletal status (Genant *et al.* 1996; Grampp *et al.* 1997; Njeh *et al.* 1999). The case for wider adoption of QUS technology has been enhanced by the findings of recent prospective studies that confirm that QUS studies in the calcaneus can predict hip fractures in the elderly as effectively as DXA (Hans *et al.* 1996; Bauer *et al.* 1997; Pluijm *et al.* 1999). However, further studies are needed to examine whether QUS is effective at predicting fracture risk in younger women (Thompson *et al.* 1998). One important advantage of DXA has been the stability of calibration of equipment in the clinical environment. In contrast, in the authors' experience, some early-generation QUS systems have shown significant technical problems due to instrumental drift, a problem that is compounded by the lack of suitable anthropomorphic phantoms for monitoring stability. Notwithstanding these problems, QUS technology clearly has an extremely promising future with the potential to make bone densitometry studies much more widely available, and it is probable that its use for routine clinical studies will expand greatly within the next few years.

New developments in scan interpretation

The new developments in equipment for bone densitometry are leading to a more critical examination of how scan findings should be interpreted. Although the WHO task group definition of osteoporosis has proved suitable for spine, hip and forearm BMD measurements, there is no reason to think that the same threshold T-score of -2.5 is appropriate for BMD measurements at other sites in the skeleton or for alternative technologies such as QUS (Faulkner *et al.* 1999). One issue is that the rate of change of BMD differs at different skeletal sites depending on the proportion of trabecular and cortical bone and their different rates of turnover at different sites. Another difficulty with T-scores is the choice of the population SD as a basis for normalising BMD changes when this measure reflects not only real differences between individuals' skeletal status, but also includes unavoidable measurement errors such as those due to heterogeneity in bone marrow and soft tissue composition affecting DXA (Svendsen *et al.* 1995) and diffraction and phase cancellation errors affecting QUS (Petley *et al.* 1995). The difficulties of basing scan interpretation on T-scores can be illustrated by plotting reference data for different BMD sites and for QUS expressed in T-score units (Figure 2.3). In this way it becomes obvious that T-score changes due to ageing and the menopause occur at different rates for some measurements compared with others and that these differences may be particularly significant for certain QUS devices.

The issues discussed above are leading to revised concepts for the interpretation of scan results (Gluer and Hans 1999). One method of ensuring greater equivalence between different types of measurement is to define thresholds for treatment recommendations for different devices based on identifying the lowest quartile of the

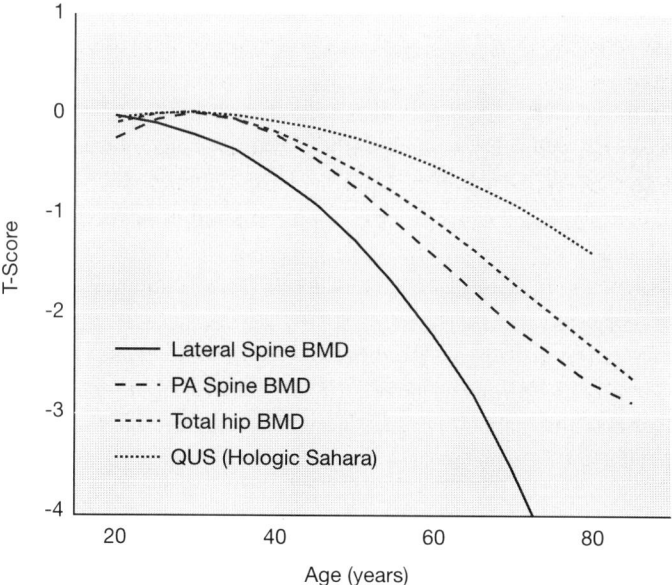

Figure 2.3 Age-related decline in mean T-score for white female subjects for different BMD measurement sites and for a quantitative ultrasound device (Hologic Sahara) (sources of reference data: lateral and PA spine BMD: Hologic Inc manufacturer's normative data (Kelly 1990); total hip BMD: NHANES study (Looker *et al.* 1998)]; QUS: (Frost *et al.* 1999)

elderly population, say between age 65 and 75. When combined with studies to establish young adult reference data, such data would generate for each device a T-score threshold equivalent to the WHO definition of osteoporosis. Beyond this, in a longer term development, equipment might be calibrated to interpret scan results in terms of fracture risk rather than T-scores, thus ensuring that there is an equivalent basis for treatment decisions whatever type of technology is employed.

Is one type of measurement superior to the rest?

Considerations such as those discussed above lead back to the fundamental issue of whether some types of measurement are inherently superior to others. This question is prompted in part by the weak to moderate correlations reported for BMD measurements in different regions of the skeleton ($r \approx 0.6$ to 0.8) or between QUS and BMD measurements ($r \approx 0.4$ to 0.6) (Grampp *et al.* 1997). As a consequence, when treatment decisions are based on thresholds such as the WHO definition of osteoporosis, different individuals may be selected for treatment based on different types of measurement. As a result, some investigators have advocated that measurements on peripheral devices such as forearm DXA or QUS should be used to make treatment decisions only for those patients with very low or very high results, with borderline cases being referred for a definitive diagnosis based on conventional spine and hip DXA (Baran *et al.* 1997). It is therefore important to examine critically the widespread belief that some types of measurement are more reliable than others.

The nature of the decisions about treatment for osteoporosis based on bone densitometry measurements can be understood by reference to the receiver operating characteristic (ROC) diagram plotted in Figure 2.4. This shows on the horizontal axis the percentage of patients referred for assessment who are recommended for preventive treatment of osteoporosis based on the chosen threshold. Of the patients scanned a certain subgroup will eventually sustain a fracture. The vertical axis in Figure 2.4 shows the percentage of patients in the fracture subgroup who are included in the treatment group plotted as a function of the odds ratio of the measurement technique. Any treatment policy (T-scores, lowest quartile, fracture risk) based on any type of measurement (spine, hip or forearm BMD or QUS) amounts to selecting an operating point on this plot. The higher the OR figure, the larger the percentage of patients who later suffer a fracture who are recommended for treatment. For example, if a decision is made to treat the lowest 25 per cent of patients, Figure 2.4 shows that for odds ratios of 1.5, 2.0, 2.5 and 3.0 the proportion of fracture patients treated is 39 per cent, 51 per cent, 60 per cent and 66 per cent respectively. According to the choice of BMD site or measurement technology, different individuals may be included in the group of future fracture patients who get treated. The only basis for preferring one type of measurement rather than another is that it has a higher OR figure. There is therefore a case that, based on present knowledge, hip BMD is the optimum measurement (Figure 2.2). However, the margin of advantage is small and is in any

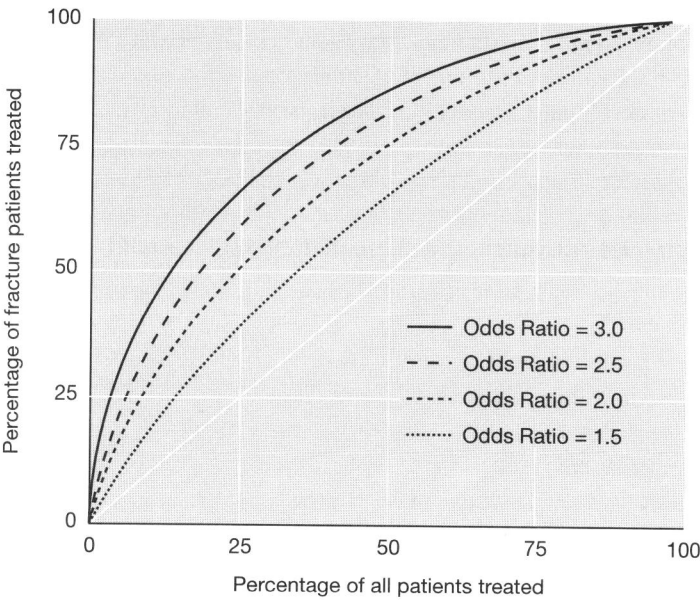

Figure 2.4 Curves for different odds ratios relating: (i) on the horizontal axis: the percentage of patients referred for assessment who are below the chosen threshold for recommending preventive treatment for osteoporosis; (ii) on the vertical axis: the percentage of patients who will sustain a future fragility fracture whose BMD is below the treatment threshold. For example, if a decision is made to treat all patients in the lowest quartile of BMD, the treatment group will include 39 per cent, 51 per cent, 60 per cent and 66 per cent of future fracture cases for odds ratios of 1.5, 2.0, 2.5 and 3.0 respectively. The higher the odds ratio, the more successful a measurement site or technology is at identifying those patients who will later have a fracture (data from Blake *et al.* 1999)

case obscured by the statistical errors in the evaluations of odds ratios. A simpler, cheaper and more widely available technology such as QUS might therefore be preferable, especially given that any disadvantage in terms of the odds ratio could be compensated by a small adjustment of the treatment threshold in Figure 2.4. However, the above remark requires some qualification since it cannot be assumed that all QUS devices have OR figures of around 2.0 (Hans *et al.* 1996; Bauer *et al.* 1997) and some models may be significantly better than others.

Conclusion

Great advances have taken place in the past decade in making equipment for bone densitometry more widely available. Better information is available on the effectiveness of BMD and QUS measurements for predicting fracture risk and the efficacy of treatments for preventing fractures, while the WHO Task Group definition of osteoporosis has provided a rationale for scan interpretation. Equally, a great deal remains to be achieved before all the potential benefits of DXA and QUS are fully realised. These include wider acceptance of the role of measurement techniques for the peripheral skeleton, especially their extension into primary care, and better information on the comparative advantages of different measurement sites and different technologies. Especially important is the development of new guidelines for scan interpretation designed to facilitate decisions over patient treatment and which put these on a consistent basis for measurements at different sites and using different technologies.

References

Baran DT, Faulkner KG, Genant HK *et al.* (1997) Diagnosis and management of osteoporosis: guidelines for the utilization of bone densitometry. *Calcif Tissue Int* **61**, 433–440.

Barlow DH (1994). *Report of the Advisory Group on Osteoporosis.* Department of Health, London.

Bauer D, Gluer C-C, Cauley *et al.* (1997). Broadband ultrasonic attenuation predicts fractures strongly and independently of densitometry in older women. *Arch Intern Med* **157**, 629–634.

Black D, Cummings SR, Genant HK *et al.* (1992) Axial and appendicular bone density predict fractures in older women. *J Bone Miner Res* **7**, 633–638.

Black DM, Cummings SR, Karpf DB *et al.* (1996). Randomised trial of effect of alendronate on risk of fracture in women with existing vertebral fractures. *Lancet* **348**, 1535–1541.

Blake GM, Wahner HW, Fogelman I (1999). *The Evaluation of Osteoporosis: Dual Energy X-ray Absorptiometry and Ultrasound in Clinical Practice.* Martin Dunitz, London.

Chapuy MC, Arlot ME, Duboeuf F *et al.* (1992). Vitamin D_3 and calcium to prevent hip fractures in elderly women. *N Engl J Med* **327**, 1637–1642.

Consensus development conference (1993) Diagnosis, prophylaxis and treatment of osteoporosis. *Am J Med* **94**, 646–650.

Cummings SR, Black DM, Nevitt MC *et al.* (1993) Bone density at various sites for prediction of hip fractures. *Lancet* **341**, 72–75.

Delmas PD, Bjarnason NH, Mitlak BH *et al.* (1997). Effects of raloxifene on bone mineral density, serum cholesterol concentrations, and uterine endometrium in post-menopausal women. *N Engl J Med* **337**, 1641–1647.

Eastell R (1998). Treatment of post-menopausal osteoporosis. *N Engl J Med* **338**, 736–746.

Faulkner KG, von Stetten E, Miller P (1999). Discordance in patient classification using T-scores. *J Clin Densiometry* **2**, 343–350.

Frost ML, Blake GM, Fogelman I (1999). Contact quantitative ultrasound: an evaluation of precision, fracture discrimination, age-related bone loss and applicability of the WHO criteria. *Osteoporosis Int* **10**, 441–449.

Genant HK, Engelke K, Fuerst T *et al.* (1996). Noninvasive assessment of bone mineral and structure: state of the art. *J Bone Miner Res* **11**, 707–730.

Gluer C-C & Hans D (1999). How to use ultrasound for risk assessment: a need for defining strategies. *Osteoporosis Int* **9**, 193–195.

Grampp S, Genant HK, Mathur A *et al.* (1997). Comparisons of non-invasive bone mineral measurements in assessing age-related loss, fracture discrimination and diagnostic classification. *J Bone Miner Res* **12**, 697–711.

Hans D, Dargent-Molina P, Schott A *et al.* (1996). Ultrasonographic heel measurements to predict hip fracture in elderly women: the EPIDOS prospective study. *Lancet* **348**, 511–514.

Hui SL, Slemenda CW, Johnston CC (1988). Age and bone mass as predictors of fracture in a prospective study. *J Clin Invest* **81**, 1804–1809.

Kanis JA, Delmas P, Burckhardt P *et al.* (1997). Guidelines for the diagnosis and management of osteoporosis. *Osteoporosis Int* **7**, 390–406.

Kelly TL (1990). Bone mineral density reference databases for American men and women. *J Bone Miner Res* **5**(Suppl 1), S249.

Looker AC, Wahner HW, Dunn WL *et al.* (1998). Updated data on proximal femur bone mineral levels of US adults. *Osteoporosis Int* **8**, 468–489.

Marshall D, Johnell O, Wedel H (1996). Meta-analysis of how well measures of bone mineral density predict occurrence of osteoporotic fractures. *Br Med J* **312**, 1254–1259.

Melton LJ, Atkinson EJ, Cooper C *et al.* (1999) Vertebral fractures predict subsequent fractures. *Osteoporosis Int* **10**, 214–221.

Njeh CF, Fuerst T, Hans D *et al.* (1999). Radiation exposure in bone mineral density measurement. *Appl Radiat Isotopes* **50**, 215–236.

Njeh CF, Hans D, Fuerst T, Gluer C-C, Genant HK (1999). *Quantitative Ultrasound: Assessment of Osteoporosis and Bone Status.* Martin Dunitz, London.

Petley GW, Robins PA, Aindow JD (1995). Broadband ultrasonic attenuation: are current measurement techniques inherently inaccurate? *Br J Radiol* **68**, 1212–1214.

Pluijm SMF, Graafmans WC, Bouter LM, Lips P (1999). Ultrasound measurements for the prediction of osteoporotic fractures in elderly people. *Osteoporosis Int* **9**, 550–556.

Reid IR (1997). Preventing glucocorticoid-induced osteoporosis. *N Engl J Med* **337**, 420–421.

Svendsen OL, Hassager C, Skodt V *et al.* (1995). Impact of soft tissue on in-vivo accuracy of bone mineral measurements in the spine, hip and forearm: a human cadaver study. *J Bone Miner Res* **10**, 868–873.

Thompson PW, Taylor J, Oliver R, Fisher A (1998). Quantitative ultrasound (QUS) of the heel predicts wrist and osteoporosis-related fractures in women age 45–75 years. *J Clin Densitom* **1**, 219–225.

World Health Organization (1994). *Assessment of Fracture Risk and its Application to Screening for Post-menopausal Osteoporosis.* WHO Technical Report Series 843. WHO, Geneva.

PART 2

Investigation and assessment of osteoporosis in primary and secondary care

Chapter 3

Osteoporosis: a primary care perspective

Allan L Harris

Introduction

Osteoporosis has been called the 'silent epidemic' (Cooper & Melton 1992). There is a huge burden of mortality and morbidity in the population with 200,000 fractures annually in the United Kingdom. This is estimated to cost the National Health Service (NHS) £940 million a year (London *et al.* 1999). For the conceivable future, each Health Authority is going to be faced each year with increasing demands on its resources from escalating costs of treating osteoporotic fractures in an ageing population as well as the increasing costs of prevention (Anonymous 1999).

There is no consensus that general population screening for osteoporosis is either cost effective or appropriate (Fogelman 1999) but there is scope in general health promotion activities of Primary Health Care Teams to emphasise the importance of general health measures which may reduce the future possibility of developing osteoporosis. The National Osteoporosis Society has produced a strategy for Primary Care Groups (*Accidents, Falls, Fractures and Osteoporosis*, December 1999) (Cooper *et al.* 1999) which gives an 'Action Plan for Population-Wide Primary Prevention Measures'.

The main thrust of primary care intervention should be directed at identifying those patients with established disease as well as those patient groups at the highest risk of developing osteoporosis. There should be structures in place in practices to avoid patients who have the disease, or who are very likely to develop it, slipping through the net and not being treated. A high-risk case-finding strategy was recommended by the Royal College of Physicians in their report *Osteoporosis. Clinical Guidelines for Prevention and Treatment* (London *et al.* 1999).

Awareness of osteoporosis by the primary care team

Osteoporosis is a condition that is ideally suited for management in primary care. It is a chronic condition, with late clinical consequences, preventable in the early stages, identifiable with appropriate screening and investigation. It is a condition where long-term surveillance and treatment is required. Primary care teams have considerable experience of managing chronic diseases and already have chronic disease systems in place for their practice populations. Prevention is a key role of the primary care team. At present there is no requirement to provide care in a systematic manner for osteoporosis as there is, for example, in diabetes and asthma. There are practices that have, in recent years, expanded their prevention and treatment role to other areas, most notably to cardiovascular disease, with no formal financial inducements as there have been for diabetes and asthma. Professional awareness and interest in quality has driven these changes as well as good evidence being widely publicised from well-conducted clinical trials. Osteoporosis can achieve the same profile of importance by a process of education and informing the professional groups involved.

All members of the primary care team in direct patient contact, such as GPs, practice nurses, health visitors, physiotherapists, occupational therapists, should have an awareness of the importance of osteoporosis. There should be an agreed practice protocol for investigation and treatment of appropriate patients.

Practice nurses are an important professional group dealing with individuals at high risk of rapid bone loss, especially women at and around the menopause. Nurses are generally better than doctors at following management guidelines and patients already routinely receive health education interventions from nurses. There would be scope for continuing professional development of nurses in this area to improve their knowledge of osteoporosis. Increased patient education might then be effective in improving concordance with medical treatment, especially continuation of HRT, as well as increasing the adoption of lifestyle changes.

Osteoporosis is common, there is a good evidence base for interventions but its management in general practice tends to be piecemeal and lacks the direction that we have achieved for other chronic diseases. It is the belief of the author that we lack a common strategy for tackling this problem, possibly because the messages from guidelines have not been implemented, but also because of the insidious nature of the disease.

One of the major obstacles to any effective disease management in primary care must be the pressure of increasing workload that diverts us away from taking the longterm view to dealing with the pressures of the present. It is too easy for the demands of the presenting symptom to relegate prevention and case-finding in the consultation. Shortage of time is one of the great constraints in primary care. We have had steadily increasing clinical and administrative work placed upon us by central government as well as by a more aware and demanding public in recent years. Numbers of consultations rise year on year and the consultation itself has become more complex.

Audit systems can perform some of the tasks of identifying patients in at-risk groups. This requires resourcing for the task to be performed effectively, as audit is a very time-consuming activity. Operating a call and recall system is expensive both in administrative time and professional input and cannot simply be added onto an already strained system. Although the Government has identified osteoporosis as a priority area in *Our Healthier Nation* (Department of Health 1998) so far there has been little central guidance as to how we should place osteoporosis identification and treatment among other demands. Although accident prevention, including falls in the elderly, is one of the targets in *Our Healthier Nation* the document gives only general pointers as to how this might be achieved. Cardiovascular disease and cancers are the current areas that are attracting most funding and political direction. If osteoporosis is to be given the importance it undoubtedly should have, then adequate resources will have to be allocated to it.

The role of guidelines

General practitioners have been provided with guidelines in the detection and management of osteoporosis, including those of the Primary Care Rheumatology Society (PCR) who produced their 'minimum acceptable' guidelines within the last year. These particular guidelines were deliberately condensed onto a double side of laminated A4 paper. It was decided that anything more comprehensive, although more informative, would fail as it would not be referred to in the consultation. The Royal College of Physicians guidelines (1999) although comprehensive and clear are not suitable for use in the consultation but are a useful resource for a practice library. The College does however have a summary of its guidelines available on laminated sheets and these are more suitable for use in the consultation room. They can be accessed on the Internet, as can the summary of their recommendations (www.doh.gov.uk/osteop.htm). The National Osteoporosis Society has also produced educational materials and guidelines suitable for use in primary care and their website is also a useful resource (www.nos.org.uk). For a more international set of recommendations the web-site of the National Osteoporosis Foundation in the USA is worth visiting (www.nof.org).

We don't know how widely any guidelines are actively used in everyday practice. For them to be useful and used they have to be immediately accessible, clear and unambiguous. The key to increased use of guidelines must be accessibility. They have to be relatively straightforward for immediate use in the consultation. They have to be relevant to general practitioners, they have to be evidence based, and they have to be realistic. Somerset Local Medical Committee has developed criteria for assessing guidelines for general practice, which may become more widely accepted. (Yoxhall 2000). The use of computers in general practice has increased in recent years and it is stated government policy that all GPs will eventually be linked to NHS Net which it is intended will give GPs access to high quality information in the consultation, where it is needed. Extension of the PRODIGY prescribing advice and guidance scheme is being encouraged by government in an attempt to rationalise GP prescribing. The provision of guidelines electronically at the desktop, in the consultation, could improve the management of many diseases but not without costs of time and resources in developing these. In the author's own practice, a practice based Intranet has been developed, which gives partners access to our formulary guidelines, common disease protocols, and so on at the click of a mouse, easily accessible in consultations.

There may well be an increasing knowledge base in practice but some of the clearest evidence of increased clinical activity has to be the escalating costs of pharmaceutical products for the treatment of osteoporosis in general practice. Some of this increase in prescribing is due to pharmaceutical companies being active in promoting their products and using some of the available clinical evidence in a competitive marketplace. Some prescribing is probably inappropriate and some drugs are very expensive. Advice to General Practitioners as to the most cost-effective way to prescribe must be part of a PCG wide initiative in managing the disease. (Torgerson 1999.) We are still under-treating this condition and it seems likely that costs are going to continue to rise in the future. In an era of cost limited drug budgets doctors will need guidance as to the most effective and economical way to treat osteoporosis. The best evidence of treatment which is effective both in reducing the burden of disease and in avoiding costs of treating the fractures prevented is essential for rational prescribing.

There is evidence from independent authorities on the most appropriate interventions available in certain groups of patients. (Chapuy *et al.* 1992; Pols *et al.* 1999). This may have changed some prescribing behaviour. Bandolier, the Oxford based evidence based medicine periodical and website have produced some illuminating meta-analyses in recent years on osteoporosis that have been widely distributed through general practice. This information is accessible, readable and addresses GPs in language with which they are familiar, especially the concept of 'numbers needed to treat.'

Diagnosis and difficulties in primary care

The World Health Organisation (WHO) (1994) agreed a definition of osteoporosis that is accepted internationally:

'A progressive systemic skeletal disease characterised by low bone mass and micro-architectural deterioration of bone tissue, with a consequent increase in bone fragility and susceptibility to fracture'.

One of the greatest virtues of the current relationship of GP and patient in the United Kingdom is the continuity of care provided. The doctor will be familiar with his patient and should recognise changes that occur over long periods of time. Chronic conditions can appear so slowly however that the diagnosis is only immediately obvious to the doctor unfamiliar with the patient. Hypothyroidism is the classic diagnosis made by the new doctor seeing the patient for the first time. Osteoporosis can be missed through familiarity. Both patients and doctors expect some shrinking as part of ageing but excessive amounts of height loss may be accepted when they are in fact pathological and preventable.

Diagnosis can be difficult in an insidious condition until an 'event' occurs, which may be as subtle as noting a painless loss in height over time, or as dramatic as a fractured hip. The importance of case-finding prior to these events occurring, in other words finding asymptomatic patients at high risk of developing disease, should be an important way of reducing the burden of osteoporosis for the future. Identifying such patients and then persuading them that they may need to think about lifestyle changes and possibly treatment longterm will represent an increased practice workload, (though opportunistic case-finding may occur.) Screening the practice database for risk factor information, which will not have been collected systematically before since there has been no requirement to do so as a Health Promotion exercise, could be unprofitable. Better recording of risk factor information would be a necessary first step to a high risk screening programme but although the risk factors for the disease are well known (Cummings *et al.* 1995), there has been no systematic effort made to record these in primary care. The former Health Promotion Schemes of the 1990s did lead to some baseline information being recorded for height and weight on large numbers of patients. The author has found it helpful, as part of the process leading to diagnosis, to have this information available in a number of patients. Some loss of height is inevitable as part of the normal ageing process but more extreme differences point to the need to investigate.

Elderly patients frequently have a complicated agenda in the consultation. Multiple pathologies co-exist. Medication regimes in the older patient are complicated. Concordance with treatment may be affected both by complex multiple drug regimes, side effects of drugs and problems of communication and comprehension. The incidence of osteoporosis rises as we age, in both sexes, and the numbers of potential patients in the over 80 age groups who might benefit from treatment is huge.

Younger patients, particularly at the time of the menopause, may feel little incentive to take treatment to treat a risk of developing future disease when they have no present symptoms. Hormone replacement therapy (HRT) is more likely to be taken for the symptoms of the menopause. It is important to take the opportunity of consultation to counsel and educate the patient fully, taking more than a limited gynaecological approach but to include all aspects of health care so that the longer term benefits, including those on the skeleton are understood. (Kleerekoper 1998). There is increasing evidence that HRT provides benefit in the 'current account', bone loss accelerating again when treatment stops, even though some longterm benefit accrues. (Michaëlsson *et al.* 1998.)

A normal diagnostic assessment in general practice will include clinical history taking and examination, basic biochemistry, (to include full blood count, erythrocyte sedimentation rate, liver function tests, serum calcium and alkaline phosphatase.) The biochemical assessment is more to exclude important secondary causes of osteoporosis than to establish the primary diagnosis.

Standard radiography, performed for other purposes, may show vertebral deformity due to osteoporotic fracture but a more common incidental observation by the radiographer is osteopenia. By the time that osteopenia is radiologically apparent 20–30 per cent of the total bone mass has been lost. Low bone mineralisation in a patient, discovered incidentally on x-ray, can be a useful diagnostic clue that osteoporosis is likely. It should be one of the triggers suggesting the need for further assessment of the patient.

The low impact fracture is a common 'endpoint', which can make the practitioner aware that the patient has developed osteoporosis. However, by this stage we have lost significant opportunity to prevent morbidity and mortality by primary prevention. For each GP, the occurrence of an osteoporotic fracture in an individual patient is a relatively uncommon event (200,000 fractures/35,000 GPs = approximately six per year). The silent incidence of vertebral osteoporotic fracture is probably considerable, possibly in excess of 48,000 fractures annually (Cooper & Melton 1992), and this may be an underestimate.

The fracture is a marker of risk, certainly a very important indicator that this patient is at significant risk of future fracture and most GPs would regard a low impact fracture as diagnostic of osteoporosis. Hopefully this should lead to intervention. Since they are relatively infrequent, these patients should be readily identified, investigated and treated. Experience shows that this is not always the case and years may elapse before any preventative treatment starts. The spur to intervention may be a further fracture but the GP and the orthopaedic specialist may miss even the significance of this. The patient may have a clear history of several fractures over several years, clear evidence of height loss and the development of a thoracic kyphosis and still remain untreated for osteoporosis even when they present to the doctor with other complaints.

Dual energy x-ray absorptiometry (DXA) scanning

The 'gold-standard' investigation to establish the diagnosis of osteoporosis is DXA scanning. With every reduction of 1 standard deviation in bone density there is a 2–2.5 fold increase in the likelihood of fracture. The WHO definition of osteoporosis as a T score at the spine or hip, <-2.5 has become widely accepted. (Fogelman 1999; Genant et al. 1999).

There are approximately 110 DXA machines in this country but their distribution is variable. Open access by GPs to this investigation is not universal. The machines are not all working at their full capacity, which is a poor use of capital resources. It has been estimated (Cooper et al. 1999) that a PCG of 100,000 population should require 1,000 DXA scans a year. The basic figure of 1,000 scans per 100,000 population would suggest a need for 560,000 scans annually for the country, 5,000 scans per machine. For a GP list of 1,800 this would equate to 18 scans per GP annually. The criteria for ordering scans vary around the country, some units being quite restrictive and setting detailed criteria before GPs can order one, other areas only allowing scans after consultant opinion, some areas being quite liberal in the freedom with which GPs can order these investigations. (Personal information obtained from GP UK, the general practice on-line discussion group.) The average cost of a DXA scan is around £45, the cost of one month's treatment with the most expensive drug used routinely in treatment of osteoporosis, Alendronate, is £23.12 per 28 days, £301.38 annually. Before embarking on longterm and expensive treatment it is surely necessary, where doubt exists, to establish the need for it.

Other diagnostic tools are available to GPs to aid in the diagnosis of osteoporosis but so far none has been as well validated as DXA scanning.

Ultrasound scanning has been shown to provide good evidence of risk of future fracture (Reid 1998; Fogelman 1999). There is no accepted standard as yet for this investigation, since there are many different machines with different characteristics, not all being comparable. Therefore, ultrasound cannot, at present, give more than an indication of risk. Ultrasound cannot establish the diagnosis of osteoporosis but it does give a valuable indication of which patients should go onto DXA scanning. (Garnero *et al.* 1998). The main advantage of ultrasound to the general practitioner could be as a screening tool for further investigation. The devices are suitable for use by trained staff in the primary care setting but the capital costs of equipment and the numbers of patients who would need screening in each individual practice would make purchase by a Primary Care Group (PCG) as part of an osteoporosis strategy the most economic approach to provision of this service.

Biochemical markers of bone formation (serum osteocalcin and bone specific alkaline phosphatase) and bone resorption markers (urine N- and C-terminal telopeptides) are superficially an extremely attractive way for GPs to investigate osteoporosis as they could provide a quick way of determining bone turnover and response to treatment. However there are so far no standard tests or sets of references for GPs to use and so these investigations remain on the horizon for use by GPs. If the tests could be standardised they would represent a valuable aid to diagnosis and treatment response. We lack the skills to interpret the results and the potential variability of the individual result makes repeated measurements necessary. The future potential of such investigations is considerable, especially in monitoring response to treatment (Rosen *et al.* 1998).

Risk factors

Investigation is appropriate only in cases when it will change management. It is reasonable to treat on clinical grounds when the diagnosis is unequivocal, especially when there is restricted access to confirmatory investigations. This is consistent with much activity in general practice, where judgements about when to start treatment are frequently empirical and based on clinical grounds.

If a woman decides that she would like to take HRT for symptomatic relief of menopausal symptoms, her bone density does not have to enter into the equation. Knowledge of her bone mineral density might however influence her decision as to whether she will take, and continue, the treatment longterm. Most women do not take HRT for years as their primary motivation is symptom relief and their fear is the increased risk of breast cancer with long term usage. A DXA bone mineral density might be important in helping her to come to a decision on continuing treatment but has no part to play in the decision to treat for symptom relief. Education and support can influence improved uptake and continuance of treatment (Coope & Coope 1996; Purdie *et al.* 1996; Steel *et al.* 1998; Jamal *et al.* 1999).

In an ideal world we would establish the diagnosis of osteoporosis beyond doubt prior to treatment but where investigations are rationed, either by non-availability or long waiting times, this may not be practicable. There is an element of false economy in this approach as the available treatments vary widely in price and all have to be continued longterm. It would probably be cost-effective to focus on patients who need treatment and exclude patients who would not be at high risk of developing osteoporosis in the future.

There are clearly groups of patients at increased risk of fracture who need treatment, whether investigations are available or not (PCR 1999):

- Low oestrogen states: early menopause, <45 years (particularly for those women who have a surgical menopause after hysterectomy and bilateral salpingo-oophorectomy)
- Previous osteoporotic fractures, radiographic evidence of osteopenia or vertebral deformity, loss of height and the development of thoracic kyphosis. A definite history of low impact fracture is almost certainly going to be associated with osteoporosis. It may, in a well resourced system, make sense to obtain a baseline DXA scan (London et al. 1999). However, a fracture is more likely to influence the general practitioner to treatment than the availability of DXA scanning.
- Prolonged corticosteroid use, over 7.5mgs daily for months, (the National Osteoporosis Society (NOS) consensus was for six months' continuous usage in their Guidance document (Reid et al. 1998)) requires measures to protect the skeleton from the effects of these drugs. It is possible that there could be a risk of future litigation against GPs who fail to counsel their patients about the risks of osteoporosis after taking steroids longterm and their need for prophylactic treatment. The PCR judged that it is an essential part of steroid therapy that bone preserving treatment should be offered and that this should be documented in the notes.

There are other groups of patients in whom there is an increased likelihood of developing osteoporosis and in whom it is appropriate to investigate to establish risk or to establish a baseline from which the effectiveness of treatment can be judged:

- A history of over 12 months amenorrhea, whether due to excessive exercise, anorexia nervosa or other secondary ovarian under-activity
- Low body mass index <19kg/m^2
- Family history of osteoporosis or osteoporotic fracture
- Secondary osteoporosis to other diseases occurs including chronic renal failure, coeliac disease and other malabsoption syndromes, hyperthyroidism, Cushing's syndrome, hyperparathyroidism, hypogonadism (especially in males), prolonged immobilisation, post transplantation. In most of these clinical situations there will

be an involvement of secondary care specialists where appropriate investigations should be readily available

- Patients with a low calcaneal qualitative ultrasound result are at higher risk of having osteoporosis. It appears that ultrasound is an excellent predictive risk factor for osteoporosis even if the actual result may not be diagnostic of osteoporosis.

The majority of patients who present with clinical features of osteoporosis will fit within these categories. Risk factors are an important part of the clinical assessment of the patient and can assist in diagnosis, but the most important factor for the professional is an awareness of the disease.

Which treatment strategy should the GP recommend?

Lifestyle

General practitioners and practice nurses have an increasing role in advising patients about changes in behaviour that can modify the risks of diseases. We should be advising all patients to stop smoking, one of the modifiable risk factors for osteoporosis as for so much else, increasing weight bearing exercise, having an adequate intake of calcium, obtaining sufficient exposure to sunlight for Vitamin D synthesis, avoiding excess alcohol intake. We should be encouraging young people, especially women, to have an adequate diet, rich in calcium, and to take weight bearing exercise. Our role is to inform the patient so that they can make appropriate choices. If there is added weight to our advice supported by bone mineral density assessment this may improve the adoption of healthier lifestyle.

Prevention of falls in the elderly

This is a potential way of reducing fractures, especially in dependent patients in institutions. The measures suggested in Anonymous (1999) include looking at prescribed drugs, exercise, visual problems and providing hip protector pants. Accident prevention, as part of the *Our Healthier Nation* initiative is going to be a PCG priority. Evidence-based measures that can be shown to be effective in reducing falls will become a priority for implementation.

Medication

Hormone replacement therapy has been shown to be effective in the prevention of osteoporosis in women and has been used for many years. Most HRT use in general practice is prescribed for symptom relief at and around the time of the menopause. There has been increased awareness among patients of the benefits of HRT and there is increased tendency for treatment to be continued longterm in some patients, not necessarily for reasons of bone preservation or cardiovascular benefit, but because they feel generally better taking the treatment. An important factor increasing the take-up and continuation of HRT has been the formulation in recent years of 'no-bleed' continuous combined preparations that are more acceptable to the patient. Tibolone is an alternative form of HRT which, if used in women several years after the menopause, can give effective symptom relief as well as little in the way of menstruation. However, as with the continuous combined tablets, some initial bleeding can occur. Tibolone also produces significant increases in bone density. It has always been easier to get patients who have had hysterectomy to continue treatment with unopposed oestrogen because they appreciate the need to replace oestrogen without having the inconvenience of continued menstruation.

The major concern of patients regarding longterm use of HRT is the increased risk of breast cancer, which, although small in absolute terms, is real and is deemed unacceptable by many patients.

There is evidence that calcium and vitamin D are deficient in much of the elderly population and that supplementation with these at adequate dose does reduce the incidence of fracture. Reductions in the cost of combined preparations have been seen in recent months. These supplements are generally well tolerated and acceptable to the patient.

A study by Chapuy *et al.* (1992) of elderly patients in institutions did show benefit from treatment with vitamin D and calcium and this might suggest the need to look at similar patients in a practice population. These patients are at greater risk of falls and subsequent fractures and so should be targeted. It might well be more cost effective for them to have an injection of vitamin D with their autumnal influenza vaccination allied to supplementation of the diet in the nursing home than to use continuous drug regimes.

The bisphosphonates are widely used in osteoporosis prevention and treatment in general practice but they remain expensive and there are problems with side-effects of these drugs. Cyclical etidronate and alendronate are the two drugs in most common use at present. A new bisphosphonate, risedronate, is the latest drug to be released onto the UK market. There is evidence that it has a favourable side-effect profile (Harris *et al.* 1999), as well as being an effective drug. As with all treatment and prevention with drugs for osteoporosis the problems for the GP are how long to continue the medication, whether the patient is taking the medication as directed and assessment of the efficacy of treatment. As bisphosphonates are expensive it would be reasonable to perform occasional DXA scans to check for response to treatment. These would not have to be performed frequently as the change in bone density is small with treatment and there is a small variation in DXA results which would require several years to elapse between readings for a real effect to be demonstrated. There are currently no guidelines of which the author is aware regarding the frequency with which DXA scans should be repeated by GPs.

Raloxifene is the first Selective Oestrogen Receptor Modulator (SERM) and has been shown to be effective in the treatment of osteoporosis (Ettinger *et al.* 1999.) The drug has attractive features for patients, including the absence of bleeding and a possible protective effect in breast cancer. However the drug is expensive in comparison to HRT and this makes it a second line agent at present. There is not as much evidence for its use at present as the bisphosphonates, which are in the same cost bracket. A useful review for GPs on this drug, with a comprehensive overview of HRT in general is available at www.rcpe.ac.uk/public/volume29_3c.html.

The use by GPs of other drugs, including calcitriol, fluoride and calcitonin is minimal at present.

The role of the Primary Care Group

There is a requirement for a Primary Care Group-wide approach to improving their population's health in accordance with the brief remit set out in the White Paper, *Saving Lives: Our Healthier Nation* (Department of Health 1998) which includes targets for reduction of accidents. As part of this there is a hope that reduced incidence of falls might reduce fractures in the elderly population. Health Improvement Plans for localities will have to have specific aims for action to be planned, funded and implemented. The NOS report *Prevention of Osteoporosis for Primary Care Groups* could provide a framework for development of services. Osteoporosis represents a major health burden for each population, less dramatic and emotive than cardiac disease and cancers, but still of considerable importance. Local needs need to be identified, resources consumed quantified and strategies adopted to reduce the burden of osteoporosis.

Conclusion

Osteoporosis is a chronic disease affecting both sexes. It is common and produces major morbidity and mortality. It can be prevented but this requires early diagnosis and intervention. Treatment for the established condition is available but represents a missed opportunity in preventing the development of disease.

General practice should be the focal point of osteoporosis management. At present there is an increasing burden of disease because of the ageing population. Costs of treatment, both for treatment of osteoporotic fractures and prophylaxis of the condition, are escalating. Shortage of resources, both in funding for increased drug costs, adequate professional time and appropriate investigations being available to primary care, all conspire against improved management. To improve management of this disease we must improve our awareness of the condition and increase its clinical priority. We must also be made aware of the most cost effective and evidence-based treatments available for particular groups of patients. A high-risk strategy for identification of patients with established disease and those at highest risk of developing disease has to develop across Primary Care Groups.

Treatment can be both by general lifestyle advice, tailored for each age group, and by specific pharmacological interventions. General lifestyle and health promotion advice is something that primary care should be providing to all our practice populations, both opportunistically and in screening programmes.

References

Anonymous (1999). Injuries from falls are increasing in older adults. *Bandolier* **6**, 2–5. www.jr2.ox.ac.uk/Bandolier/booth/booths/bones.html.

Chapuy MC, Arlot ME, Duboeuf F *et al.* (1992). Vitamin D3 and Calcium to prevent hip fractures in elderly women. *New England Journal of Medicine* **327**, 1637–1642.

Coope JK & Coope JR (1996). HRT, a general practice approach: how to reach the most vulnerable. *Br J Clin Pract* **50**, 38–43.

Cooper C, Brown P *et al.* (1999). *Accidents, Falls, Fractures and Osteoporosis – A Strategy for Primary Care Groups and Local Health Groups.* National Osteoporosis Society Report, London.

Cooper C & Melton LJ (1992). Vertebral fractures; how large is the silent epidemic? *British Medical Journal* **304**, 793–794.

Cummings S, Nevitt M, Browner W *et al.* (1995). Risk factors for hip fracture in white women. *New England Journal of Medicine* **332**, 767–773.

Department of Health (1998). *Saving Lives: Our Healthier Nation.* London: HMSO.

Ettinger B, Black DM, Mitlak BH *et al.* (1999). Reduction of vertebral fracture risk in postmenopausal women with osteoporosis treated with Raloxifene, *JAMA* **282**, 637–645.

Fogelman I (1999). Screening for osteoporosis. *British Medical Journal* **319**, 1148–9.

Garnero P, Dargent-Molina P, Hans D *et al.* (1998). Do markers of bone resorption add to bone mineral density and ultrasonographic heel measurement for the prediction of hip fracture in elderly women? The EPIDOS Prospective study. *Osteoporosis International* **8**, 563–569.

Genant HK, Cooper C, Poor G *et al.* (1999) Interim report and recommendations of the World Health Organization task-force for osteoporosis. *Osteoporosis International* **10**, 259–264.

Harris S, Watts N, Genant H *et al.* (1999). Effects of risedronate treatment on vertebral and nonvertebral fractures in women with postmenopausal osteoporosis. *JAMA* **282**, 1344–1352.

Jamal SA, Ridout R, Chase C *et al.* (1999). Bone mineral density testing and osteoporosis education improve lifestyle behaviours in premenopausal women: a prospective study. *J Bone Mineral Research* **14**, 2143–2149.

Kleerekoper M (1998). Detecting osteoporosis. Beyond the history and physical examination. *Postgraduate Medicine* **103**, 45–7, 51–2, 62–3.

London D, Barlow D, Cooper C *et al.* (1999). *Osteoporosis – Clinical Guidelines for Prevention and Treatment.* Royal College of Physicians, Reports 4, 6 and 18, London.

Michaëlsson K, Baron JA, Farahmand BY *et al.* (1998). Hormone replacement therapy and risk of hip fracture: population based case-control study. *BMJ* **316**, 1858–1863.

Purdie DW, Steel SA, Howey S, Doherty SM (1996). The technical and logistical feasibility of population densitometry using DXA and directed HRT intervention: a 2 year prospective study. *Osteoporosis International* **Suppl. 3**, S31–S36.

Primary Care Rheumatology Society (1999). *Minimum Standard Guidelines for PCR Members (Treatment of Osteoporosis).* PCR Society Report, North Yorkshire.

Pols H, Felsenberg D, Hanley D *et al.* (1999). Multinational, placebo-controlled, randomized trial of the effects of Alendronate on bone density and fracture risk in postmenopausal women with low bone mass: results of the FOSIT study. *Osteoporosis International* **9**, 461–468.

Reid DM (1998). The use of Quantitative Ultrasound in the Management of Osteoporosis in Primary or Secondary Care, National Osteoporosis Society position statement, London.

Reid DM, Eastell R *et al.* (1998). *Guidance on the Prevention and Management of Corticosteriod Induced Osteoporosis. National Osteoporosis Society Consensus Meeting.* Bath: National Osteoporosis Society.

Rosen HN, Moses AC, Garber J *et al.* (1998). Utility of biochemical markers of bone turnover in the follow-up of patients treated with bisphosphonates. *Calcif Tissue Int* **63,** 363–368.

Steel SA, Purdie DW, Howey S (1998). A 5 year prospective trial of BMD behaviour in HRT treated and untreated perimenopausal women. *ASBMR* F265.

Torgerson D (1999). *Osteoporosis Review* **7,** 1–4.

Yoxall H (2000). Setting standards for GP guidance. *General Practitioner*, 41–2.

Chapter 4

Investigating osteoporosis in secondary care

Michael D Stone and Jane Turton

Introduction

Osteoporosis is a problem that places a huge burden upon individuals and the health service. The lifetime risk of fracture as a result of osteoporosis is 13 per cent in men and 39 per cent in women (Melton *et al.* 1992). In the UK alone, osteoporosis results in 200,000 fractures per year at an estimated cost of £940 million (Royal College of Physicians 1999). The most widely accepted method of diagnosing osteoporosis is using the technique of dual energy x-ray absorptiometry (DXA). This provides a measure of bone mineral density (BMD), with the cut off point of -2.5 SD from the young adult mean being widely accepted as a threshold for treatment (Kanis 1994; Kröger & Reeve 1998). It is known that the risk of fracture doubles for every 1 SD loss of BMD (Figure 4.1). The presentation to the physician depends to a certain extent upon the underlying cause of the disease. However, many patients first come to the attention of the bone specialist following a low trauma fracture most typically that of a hip, wrist or vertebra. In total, 2 per cent of all over 55 year olds suffer low trauma fractures each year and of these 31 per cent require hospital admission. Half of admitted patients with such fractures are over the age of 65, meaning that 1.3 per cent of all those over 65 years of age require inpatient fracture care during a single year (Johansen *et al.* 1998). Patients presenting to the bone specialist prior to their first fracture usually do so because they, or their primary care physicians, have

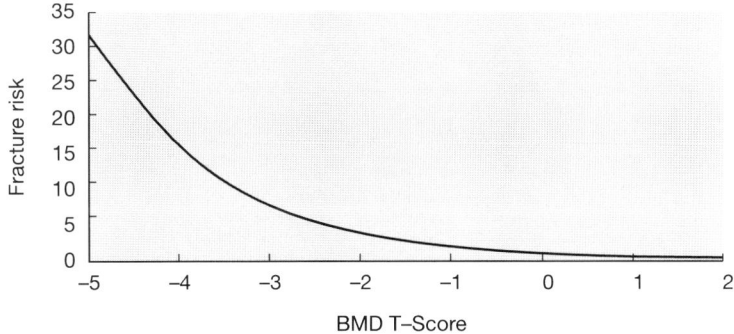

Figure 4.1 Graph showing the fracture risk relative to changes in bone density (Meunier *et al.* 1999)

identified factors which are known to predispose an individual to the development of osteoporosis.

Appropriate investigation

The appropriate investigation of osteoporosis should always follow a full history and clinical examination. As is often the case, there is an inevitable degree of overlap between primary and secondary care and referral patterns differ widely between practices. Most investigations can be requested and performed in primary care but this depends on levels of expertise, interest, time constraints and accessibility. The clinical diagnosis of osteoporosis is unreliable and the current bench mark for the diagnosis is a measurement of bone mineral density.

Dual energy x-ray absorptiometry

Duel energy x-ray absorptiometry is now the most widely accepted technique for the measurement of bone density, having been validated by large prospective cohort studies (Cummings *et al.* 1998). Most DXA scanners are centrally located in secondary care units and even mobile units are usually provided from secondary care. In Cardiff an open access service is operated for GPs whilst other centres may only accept referrals for DXA scans via an outpatient clinic. There are well-defined, nationally agreed indications for scans as well as diagnostic values (Royal College of Physicians 1999). In addition, a DXA scan enables a baseline to be established, against which the effects of treatments may be evaluated. In those individuals with osteoporosis it allows effective targeting of treatment and is probably cost-effective (Kanis *et al.* 1997). Perhaps most importantly (adopting evidence-based principles) the major inclusion criteria for the pharmacological intervention studies (randomised controlled trials with fractures as the primary outcome measure) are based on DXA measurements (Ettinger *et al.* 1999; Black *et al.* 1996). Moreover, in those patients who have bone density values above the WHO defined T-score threshold of -2.5, non-vertebral fractures are not prevented and by implication such fractures in those patients with relatively respectable bone densities may reflect risk factors independent of bone mass such as risk and mode of falling (Cummings *et al.* 1998). Significant reductions in vertebral fractures however may not be so dependent on measured DXA values (Cummings *et al.* 1998). Thus, all patients should have DXA scans prior to starting treatment, except for the frail elderly patient (Figure 4.2). In this latter group, simple supplementation with 1 gram of elemental calcium and 800 iu of vitamin D is the treatment of choice.

The use of DXA has drawbacks. The presence of some pre-existing pathologies can produce erroneous results. For example, the following conditions can produce inaccuracies in the measurement of bone density: osteomalacia, where the defect is mineralisation rather than loss of bone structure; osteoarthritis, where the bone and joint morphology may not be normal, leading to false negative results, especially in

---

Who?
- All except frail elderly

Why?
- confirms/refutes diagnosis
- clinical diagnosis is unreliable
- enables monitoring
- WHO definitions may be applied
- reference ranges are reasonably well defined
- validated technique
- probably cost-effective

Figure 4.2 The use of DXA

the spine; the presence of metal objects such as hip prostheses, previous fractures, scoliosis, obesity and previous gold therapy (Kanis *et al.* 1997).

In summary, low bone density is a good determinant of fracture risk (Compston *et al.* 1995). Although, it should not be forgotten that the aetiology of fracture is multifactorial, measurement of bone density does influence therapeutic choices, enables the physician to monitor therapy and probably aids compliance (Meunier *et al.*1999).

Establishing the differential diagnosis

Making a radiological diagnosis of osteoporosis is not sufficient, since we need to identify the patients who are at highest risk of suffering an osteoporotic fracture, and those patients for whom there is a treatable secondary underlying cause. Fifty per cent of men and 30 per cent of women with symptomatic vertebral fracture may have an underlying secondary cause (Figure 4.3) (Royal College of Physicians 1999). The investigations performed in secondary care can be tailored to the individual patient, and a more extensive range of tests should be performed for patients exhibiting symptoms or signs which raise clinical suspicion of a more sinister underlying pathology or specific secondary cause, such as unusually severe osteoporosis, young patients, obese patients, patients with unintentional weight loss and pain which does not resolve or is very severe at rest (Figure 4.4).

Radiology

Plain radiographs of the lumbar spine and/or femoral neck provide valuable information regarding the morphology of a patient's bones. Lateral lumbar spine radiographs should be performed before measurement of bone density scans in the investigation of kyphosis, loss of height and back pain to determine whether vertebral fractures are present (Kanis *et al.* 1997). Isotope bone or MRI scans may be useful in the presence of fractures to exclude metastatic bone disease.

Primary		
	Idiopathic	
	Type I post-menopausal	
	Type II age related	
Secondary		
Endocrine	hypogonadism	
	hyperparathyroidism (primary and secondary)	
	hypercortisolism (endogenous or exogenous)	
	hyperthyroidism (endogenous or exogenous)	
	hypopituitarism	
Drugs	corticosteroids	
	heparin	
	anticonvulsants	
	immunosuppressants	
Gastrointestinal	Coeliac disease	
	liver disease	
	post-gastrectomy	
	malnutrition	
Malignancy	bony metastasis	
	multiple myeloma, lymphoma, leukaemia	
	mastocytosis	
Skeletal	rheumatoid arthritis	
	ankylosing spondylitis	
	osteogenesis inperfecta	
others	pregnancy	
	Turner's syndrome	
	vitamin C deficiency	
	immobilisation	
	homocystinuria	
	renal osteodystrophy	

Figure 4.3 The classification of osteoporosis (based upon Pathy 1998)

- obese patient
- unusually severe osteoporosis
- worrying symptoms of signs such as weight loss
- unusual pattern of pain
- pain not resolving or severe
- pain at rest
- prevalent vertebral fractures
- young patients

Figure 4.4 Higher degree of clinical suspicion = more extensive tests

Haematology and biochemistry

Laboratory investigations are performed to exclude secondary causes of osteoporosis (Figure 4.3). They can also aid in the selection of treatment and set baselines for monitoring the effects of treatment.

All patients will require full blood count (FBC) and erythrocyte sedimentation rate (ESR), bone, renal and liver profiles. The extended screen (Figure 4.5) performed

All Patients
- FBC +ESR
- Bone, renal and liver profile including gamma GT

Extended Screen (most patients in secondary care)
- TFTs serum and urine immunoelectrophoresis
- serum PTH & 25(0H) vit D (esp elderly, housebound)
- 24 hour urinary calcium
- 24 hour urinary free cortisol (if Cushings suspected)
- anti-endomysial antibodies (especially if h/o anaemia, low BMI)

Men
- testosterone and SHBG

Men with vertebral fractures
- PSA

Figure 4.5 Blood and urine tests in the investigation of osteoporosis

upon most patients in secondary care also includes thyroid function tests, serum and urine immunoelectrophoresis, serum parathyroid hormone and 25(OH) vitamin D (Dawson Hughes *et al.*1997), 24 hour urinary calcium, 24 hour urinary free cortisol (if Cushing's suspected) and anti-endomysial antibodies (Selby *et al.*1999) especially if there is a history of anaemia or low BMI. In men, testosterone and SHBG should also be measured and any man presenting with vertebral fractures should have measurement of prostate specific antigen (Royal College of Physicians 1999).

Histopathology

Transiliac bone biopsy with tetracycline labelling is indicated to confirm a diagnosis of osteomalacia, in suspected hypophosphatasia, possibly in young patients and in the presence of renal osteodystrophy (Figure 4.6). If a haematological malignancy is suspected on the basis of the FBC, ESR or immunochemistry, a bone marrow aspirate will be required.

Biochemical markers

The routine use of biochemical markers in prediction of fracture is not yet justified (Meunier *et al.*1999). However, a number of specific and sensitive markers have been developed recently. These may be used to monitor both bone formation and resorption.

- young patients
- to confirm osteomalacia
- suspected hypophoshatasia
- renal osteodystrophy
- to exclude mastocytosis
- suspected haematological malignancy

Figure 4.6 Possible indications for transiliac bone biopsy

Indeed, use in a research setting suggests that they may be of particular use in the monitoring of post-menopausal bone loss, therefore improving the specificity of bone density measurement in the prediction of fracture (Garnero *et al.* 1998). There remains conflicting data on the ability of bone markers to independently predict fracture risk and their use in this context can not yet be justified (Royal College of Physicians 1999). When monitoring patients on treatment, successful treatment of osteoporosis causes a rapid decrease in bone turnover markers which correlates well with improving bone densities (Garnero & Delmas 1999).

Peripheral densitometry

Numerous devices are now commercially available for assessing bone strength at sites other than the spine and hip. Several studies have tried to determine whether the technique of calcaneal ultrasound is a reliable enough measure of bone strength to enable a clinician to safely use it in place of the more expensive and time-consuming DXA. Broad band ultrasound attenuation (BUA) and velocity seem to provide different information about bone strength compared with DXA (Njeh *et al.*1997) and can be good predictors of fracture (Hans 1999). Bone mineral density explains about 70–75 per cent of the variance in bone strength, and if BUA and velocity are combined with DXA there appears to be an increase in specificity of fracture prediction over DXA alone. There is still however insufficient data to recommend the widespread use of ultrasound alone (Glüer & Barkmann 2000). There have been difficulties in determining treatment thresholds and in defining the reference ranges and it has not yet been used in any major intervention studies. However, it is certainly better than nothing and is much cheaper than DXA.

Barriers to investigation

Bone density measurement

The initial capital outlay for, and running costs of, DXA scanners is relatively high. Hence scanners are usually located centrally in secondary care, often only in teaching centres. There is little funding allocated to the provision of scanners and many machines have been purchased on the back of research monies or charitable donations. These factors may lead to a competition for resources between primary and secondary care and long waiting times for patients. In Cardiff there are two DXA machines to which general practitioners have open access. Between November 1998 and October 1999, they performed 3,037 bone density scans, 35 per cent of which were from primary care and 65 per cent from within secondary care. Fifty seven per cent were first scans. Ultrasound densitometry would appear to be a good alternative, but the lack of validation prevents this being used as the only measure of bone density and there is no convincing data yet that it can save money by reducing the number of full DXA scans required.

Laboratory investigations

The standard haematological, biochemical and histopathological investigations are usually available in the secondary care setting. Biochemical markers are a more research orientated tool and, at present, concerns remain regarding precision of measurement, the natural diurnal variation of markers in vivo and hence the timing of samples taken (Delmas 2000). There are also issues of inter-laboratory quality control to be addressed.

Solutions

The cost-effectiveness of DXA scanning needs to be more thoroughly demonstrated in order to convince Primary Care Groups and health authorities that the availability of scanners is important. In the meantime we should target only those groups of patients at highest risk of fracture (Royal College of Physicians 1999). The methods of peripheral densitometry using ultrasound and x-ray technology need development and further validation, since portable units offer an attractive option in secondary care. More work is still required in the area of biochemical markers.

Conclusion

Although most investigations can be performed in primary care the extent to which this occurs depends on the levels of expertise, interest, time constraints and access. Consequently referral patterns differ greatly between practices. Many patients in the secondary care sector will require extensive investigations to exclude specific causes of osteoporosis or malignancy. All patients, with the exception of the frail elderly, require DXA scans. The role of biochemical markers and peripheral densitometry remains unclear.

References

Black DM, Cummings SR, Karpf DB *et al.* (1996). Randomized trial of effect of alendronate on risk of fracture in women with existing vertebral fractures. Fracture Intervention Trial Research Group. *Lancet* **384,** 1535–41.

Compston JE, Cooper C, Kanis JA (1995) Bone densitometry in clinical practice. *BMJ* 1507–10.

Compston JE & Rosen CJ (1999) *Osteoporosis. Second Edition*. London: Health Press Ltd.

Cummings SR, Black DM, Thompson DE *et al.* (1998). Effect of alendronate on risk of fracture in women with low bone density but without vertebral fractures: results from the Fracture Intervention Trial. *JAMA* **24,** 2077–82.

Dawson-Hughes B, Harris SS, Dallal GE (1997). Plasma calcidiol, season, and serum parathyroid hormone concentrations in healthy elderly men and women. *Am J Clin Nutr* **65,** 67–71.

Delmas PD (2000). The use of biochemical markers in the evaluation of fracture risk and treatment response. *Osteoporosis International* **11,** S6.

Ettinger B, Black DM, Mitlak BH *et al.* (1999). Reduction of vertebral fracture risk in postmenopausal women with osteoporosis treated with raloxifene: results from a 3-year randomized clinical trial. Multiple Outcomes of Raloxifene Evaluation (MORE) Investigators. *JAMA* **282,** 637–45.

Fogelman I (1999) Screening for osteoporosis. *BMJ* **319,** 1148–1149.

Garnero P, Dargent-Molina P, Hans D *et al.* (1998) Do markers of bone resorption add to bone mineral density and ultrasonographic heel measurement for the prediction of hip fracture in elderly women? The EPIDOS prospective study. *Osteoporosis International* **8,** 563–9

Garnero P & Delmas PD Biochemical markers of bone turnover: clinical usefulness in osteoporosis. *Ann Biol Clin* **57,** 137–48.

Glüer CC & Barkmann R (2000).Use of quantitative ultrasound in the evaluation of osteoporosis. *Osteoporosis International* **11,** S12–S14.

Hans D, Wu C, Njeh CF *et al.* (1999). Ultrasound velocity of trabecular cubes mainly reflects bone density and elasticity. *Calcif Tissue International* **64,** 18–23.

Johansen A, Evans R, Bartlett C, Stone MD (1998). Trauma admissions in the elderly: how does a patient's age affect the likelihood of their being admitted to hospital after a fracture? *Injury* **29,** 779–784.

Johansen A, Evans R.J, Stone MD *et al.* (1997). Fracture incidence in England and Wales: a study based upon the population of Cardiff. *Injury* **28,** 655–660.

Kanis JA (1994). Assessment of fracture risk and its application to screening for post-menopausal osteoporosis: synopsis of a WHO report. *Osteoporosis International* **4,** 368–81.

Kanis JA, Delmas P, Burckhardt P, Cooper C, Torgerson D (1997). Guidelines for diagnosis and management of osteoporosis. The European Foundation for Osteoporosis and Bone Disease. *Osteoporosis International* **7,** 390–406.

Kannus P, Palvanen M, Kaprio J, Parkkari J, Kroskenvuo M (1999). Genetic factors and osteoporotic fractures in elderly people: prospective 25 year follow up of a nation-wide cohort of elderly Finnish twins. *BMJ* **319,** 1334–1338.

Kröger H & Reeve J (1998). Diagnosis of osteoporosis in clinical practice. *Ann Med* **30,** 278–287.

Melton LJ III, Chrischilles EA, Cooper C, Lane AW, Riggs BL (1992) Perspective. How many women have osteoporosis? *J Bone Mineral Research* **7,** 1005–10.

Meunier PJ, Delmas PD, Eastell R *et al.* (1999). Diagnosis and management of Osteoporosis in Post menopausal Women: Clinical Guidelines. *Clinical Therapeutics* **21,** 1025–44.

Njeh CF, Boivin CM, Langton CM (1997). The role of ultrasound in the assessment of osteoporosis: a review. *Osteoporosis International* **7,** 7–22.

Pathy MSJ (1998). *Principles and Practice of Geriatric Medicine. Third Edition.* Oxford: John Wiley & Sons Ltd.

Royal College of Physicians (1999). *Osteoporosis Clinical guidelines of Prevention and Treatment.* London: Royal College of Physicians.

Selby PL, Davies M, Adams JE, Mawer EB (1999). Bone loss in celiac disease is related to secondary hyperparathyroidism. *J Bone Miner Res* **14,** 652–7.

Chapter 5

Evidence and opinion for osteoporosis prevention: new perspectives in the role of exercise, diet and hormone replacement therapy

Anne M Sutcliffe

Introduction

Osteoporosis and associated fractures are a major public health concern because they account for significant morbidity, decreased quality of life and mortality. The adverse effects of hip fractures on activities of daily living are well documented but the effects of vertebral and forearm fractures should not be underestimated. The cost of care is high and the current implications for public health expenditure are serious. There is an exponential increase in fracture incidence with age and therefore with the ageing of the population, the medical, social and economic costs of skeletal fragility are certain to grow unless effective preventive and therapeutic options can be developed. There are many possible interventions, which might decrease the risk of osteoporosis, but not all have been subjected to definitive assessment. Popular strategies, based on observational data, include dietary provision of adequate calcium throughout life, maintenance of normal body weight, avoidance of smoking and excess alcohol intake, encouragement of a physically active lifestyle, and prevention of falls in the elderly. Therapeutic interventions, which are supported by evidence from randomised controlled trials (RCT), include hormone replacement therapy (HRT) and Raloxifene in the post-menopausal woman and calcium and vitamin D supplementation in the elderly (Figure 5.1).

Prevention strategies

Ideally, the prevention of osteoporosis should include population-based and high-risk strategies. The former aims to modify an identifiable risk factor within the general population whilst the latter targets individuals at particular risk.

The population-based approach is based on the assumption that if risk factors are causally related and can be modified the impact of osteoporosis could be prevented. The common remedial factors that have been suggested include a higher level of exercise, the ingestion of a high calcium diet, and the universal use of HRT in post-menopausal women. Prevention of osteoporosis in the general population is theoretically a laudable proposition but there are several problems inherent in this approach.

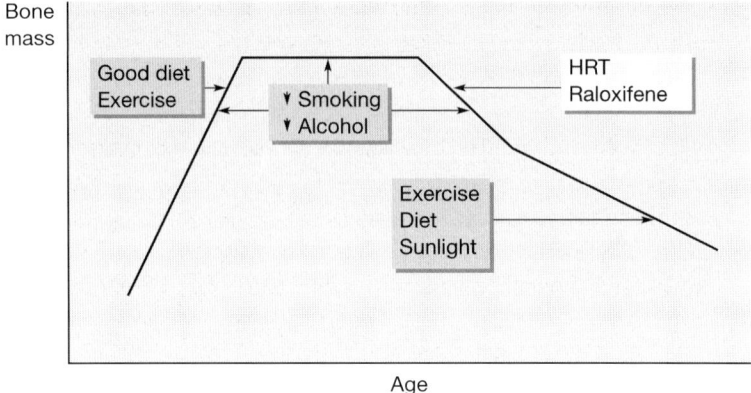

Figure 5.1 Schematic representation of lifestyle and therapeutic interventions in the prevention of osteoporosis.

All identifiable risk factors are not necessarily related to osteoporosis and, despite the high prevalence of many of these, the increase in relative risk associated with each is relatively small. A second significant problem relates to the individual's perception of health and the ability to change lifestyle habits, which may have become socially and culturally acceptable. It is also apparent that the value and feasibility of population programmes in osteoporosis prevention have never been evaluated. The high-risk approach to prevention is based on identifying those at particular risk and offering intervention. This approach assumes that high-risk individuals are easily identifiable and once identified have easy access to assessment including bone mineral density (BMD) measurements. However there are marked discrepancies between self-assessment of risk, health professionals' assessment of risk and the uniform availability of BMD measurements.

Exercise

Physical activity, particularly weight bearing exercise, provides the mechanical stimuli or 'loading' important for the maintenance and improvement of bone health, whereas physical inactivity has been implicated in bone loss and its associated health costs (Snow *et al.* 1996). The mode of impact of exercise is caused by gravitational factors or muscle pull producing strains within the skeleton, which are perceived by bone cells as osteogenic. Animal studies have demonstrated that unusual strain distributions, high strains and high strain rates seem to be particularly effective in leading to bone formation (Lanyon 1996). Application to a human model implies that strength or resistance training may have a more profound site-specific effect than endurance training. However, an endurance programme involving aerobic exercises, may also impose the necessary strains, strain rates and unusual strain distributions. The starting age of activity is important: the benefit to bone is doubled if the activity is started before or at puberty rather than after it (Kannus *et al.* 1995). In adulthood, exercise appears to largely preserve bone rather than add new bone and in the immediate post-menopausal years it is unlikely that exercise will balance the effect of oestrogen deficiency. Exercise can improve gait, balance, co-ordination, proprioception, reaction time and muscle strength in elderly people.

Many epidemiological studies have shown an association between the level of physical exercise and either bone mass or the risk of fracture and consequently the use of exercise has been advocated as a method of preventing osteoporosis. The available evidence suggests that weight bearing exercises are the more effective, but the type, degree, threshold and frequency optimal for bone mass remain uncertain. Previous literature reviews on physical activity and the relationship to osteoporosis have demonstrated inconsistent conclusions. Cross sectional studies comparing sedentary people with athletes, showed higher bone mass in the physically active groups (Snow *et al.* 1996). Cross sectional and longitudinal studies performed on post-menopausal women, however, lead to contradictory results. Krolner *et al.* (1983) demonstrated that bone mineral content of the lumbar spine was higher in active women when compared with sedentary women. Simkin *et al.* (1987) concluded that bone density was higher in active women, although their bone mineral content was unchanged after a five month exercise programme. The inconsistencies of these findings may be partly explained by the small sample sizes of published studies, differences in population characteristics, sites and outcomes studied and differences in experimental designs.

Two recent meta-analyses of the effects of physical activity have attempted to clarify and quantify the benefits of exercise on the skeleton. A meta-analysis of 18 randomised and non- randomised studies confirmed that moderate intensity exercise programmes have a beneficial effect on spinal BMD loss at the L2–4 level, in healthy post-menopausal women. However this activity was not effective for preventing forearm and femoral bone loss (Berard *et al.* 1997).

A further meta-analysis by Wolff *et al.* (1999) addressed a quantitative review of the RCTs and non randomised controlled trials (CTs) on the effects of exercise training programmes on bone mass of the lumbar spine and the femoral neck of pre- and post-menopausal women. Twenty five trials were included in the analysis and in the RCTs, exercise programmes prevented or reversed bone loss of almost 1 per cent per year compared with the controls. The overall treatment effects were consistent for the lumbar spine and the femoral neck, and also for the pre- and post-menopausal women. The overall treatment effects for the CTs were mostly twice as high as those for the RCTs, suggesting the introduction of confounding variables.

While an overall treatment effect of 0.9 per cent per year may appear small, this could have a significant impact on the development of osteoporotic fractures in large populations. Although this meta-analysis suggests that exercise training programmes may be worth considering in the prevention of osteoporosis, doubts remain about the practicalities of this approach. The beneficial effects probably persist only for the duration of exposure to exercise and the dropout rate from organised exercise programmes is high (Gleeson *et al.* 1990). The maximum length of programmes in the recent meta-analyses was two years, highlighting the need for studies of a longer duration to evaluate the feasibility and relevance of the use of exercise for bone preservation.

The vast majority of fragility fractures occur after falls. The risk of falling increases with advancing age and approximately one third of individuals over the age of 65 years falls each year. Prospective community studies have detailed risk factors for falls in elderly people and identified those old people who are likely to fall (Tinetti *et al.* 1988). The factors most commonly identified, which are possibly most amenable to interventions, are loss of muscle strength and flexibility, and impaired balance and reaction time (Myers *et al.* 1996). Meta-analysis of seven studies in the 'frailty and injuries: co-operative studies of intervention techniques' trials, showed that strength and balance training reduced the frequency of falls (Province *et al.* 1995). A recent RCT conducted in primary care in New Zealand demonstrated that a programme of strength and balance training exercises performed within the home environment significantly reduced the number of falls and injuries experienced by women aged over 80 years (Campbell *et al.* 1997). It would therefore appear that exercise training may have the potential to prevent osteoporotic fractures by simultaneously influencing multiple risk factors. Epidemiological studies show that both past and current physical activity protects against hip fracture, reducing the risk by up to 50 per cent (Joakinsen *et al.* 1997). The most appropriate combination appears to be vigorous past activity and moderate recent activity (Slemenda 1997). Weight bearing activity is most protective and some evidence suggests that even daily walking and climbing stairs may be effective (Joakinsen *et al.* 1997).

As physical exercise is readily available, relatively cheap and safe it could represent a cost-effective way of preventing osteoporosis within the general population. However, its full potential, demands lifelong adherence and acceptability, which will always be determined by the individual's specific inclination. A high-risk strategy targeted at the elderly individual at risk of falling may have a more significant impact on the reduction of falls and subsequent fractures.

Diet

The influence of nutrient intake on BMD is still largely undefined but nutritional factors are clearly of importance to bone health, as they may be modifiable. There is some evidence to suggest that calcium intake may be important during skeletal growth and peak bone mass development and supplements containing calcium and vitamin D have been shown to reduce bone loss in women and men, aged over 65 years (Dawson-Hughes *et al.* 1997). Excessive intakes of protein, sodium and caffeine are known to affect calcium metabolism but have not been shown to affect BMD adversely. The effect of intakes such as fibre, minerals and antioxidant vitamins have received little attention. The recent emergence of biologically active compounds found in various foodstuffs known as phytoestrogens has prompted in vitro and in vivo research, including effects on BMD.

Calcium

Bone is the major reservoir for calcium and the loss of calcium in later life has led to the view that adequate calcium nutrition is important for the maintenance of skeletal health. Many epidemiological studies show an association between the lifetime intake of calcium and either low bone density or a high risk of fracture in women. Conversely, many others show no such associations over a range of dietary intakes. On balance, it would appear that a higher dietary calcium intake during early childhood may have some beneficial effect on BMD, essentially maintained at the pre-pubertal stage (Lloyd *et al.* 1993). However, it is unclear whether an increased intake has any effect on skeletal consolidation or subsequent risk of fracture after longitudinal growth has ceased. Skeletal losses after the menopause may be accelerated by low calcium diets and pharmacological doses of calcium at this time may delay the rate of bone loss. Relationship between past dietary calcium intake and bone density in later life is not totally proven. However, New *et al.* (1997) have shown significant differences in BMD in pre-menopausal women (aged 45–49 years) associated with different intakes of milk in earlier life, suggesting a positive effect of calcium intake in early life on bone mass. In a large case control study of hip fracture risk in Southern Europe, exposure to a high dietary intake of calcium was associated with a significant decrease in the risk of hip fracture in both sexes. However this protective effect was confined to that 10.3 per cent of the female and 15 per cent of the male population on a low intake of calcium below the risk threshold (Johnell *et al.*1995).

It is important to recognise that past intake data are subject to recall bias and that results based on this information need to be interpreted with caution. Although uncertainties exist about the value of dietary calcium intake, high intakes are generally advocated in the population as a whole. To increase intake even further would necessitate concerted public health measures, the value and uptake of which are difficult to measure. Proposing higher dietary calcium intake in high-risk individuals may necessitate altering lifetime habits, which may prove difficult. The introduction of pharmacological calcium in these cases probably represents a more effective and feasible option.

Magnesium and potassium

In 1968, Wachmann and Bernstein hypothesised that bone mineral functions as a buffer base and the lifetime buffering of the acid load from the ingestion of mixed diets leads to gradual and accumulated bone loss. The introduction of a diet favouring 'alkaline ash' may help to limit this effect. Two nutrients, which may have such buffering effects, are potassium and magnesium, which are present in a variety of whole, unrefined foods, including fruit and vegetables. To date, relatively few studies have examined these associations but results have suggested a positive correlation between dietary intake of potassium and magnesium and improved bone status. New *et al.* (1997) found significant associations between past reported fruit intake and BMD at the spine and trochanter in pre-menopausal women. A further study in

1999 showed significant associations between intakes of potassium and magnesium and BMD (Tucker *et al.* 1999). In men these associations were seen at all hip sites and the radius and in women the associations were strongest at the trochanter. In men there appeared to be a longitudinal beneficial effect after four years. Further investigation is warranted to ascertain whether these nutrients reduce bone loss and prevent osteoporosis.

Phytoestrogens

Phytoestrogens, which are widely distributed within the plant kingdom, are functionally similar to 17 beta-oestradiol. Of particular importance to the human diet are the isoflavones and the lignans, which are found in high concentrations in legumes (soy products) and grains, cereals and linseed respectively. The growing interest in phytoestrogens is based on epidemiological data, which suggests that populations which consume phytoestrogen rich diets have a lower incidence of atherosclerotic disease, breast, endometrial and colon cancers, osteoporosis and menopausal symptoms. The incidence of osteoporosis is lower in Asian women than in their Western counterparts, and Japanese women have been reported to have a lower incidence of hip fracture than Caucasian women. Studies with phytoestrogens have largely been confined to animal models, and in rats soyabean protein has been shown to prevent bone loss by increasing formation, which then exceeded resorption (Arjmandi *et al.* 1996). Two unpublished Australian studies using soy and red clover in post-menopausal women were unable to show any effect on bone turnover after 12 weeks treatment (Mackey 1998). Several other studies have failed to show any effect on bone turnover, but a criticism of these studies would be that they were too short to observe an effect. Recent data have shown that soy intake may reduce bone loss in pre-menopausal women (Ho *et al.* 1999) and the use of isoflavone rich soy protein, over 24 weeks, also appears to limit bone loss in perimenopausal women (Alekel *et al.* 1999). Clearly, the role of phytoestrogens in osteoporosis prevention requires further investigation. From existing epidemiological evidence the incorporation of phytoestrogens in a balanced diet probably needs to be instigated at an early age, as with soy users and vegetarians, in order to confer a protective effect over a lifetime.

Hormone replacement therapy

There has been a dramatic rise in the number of hormone replacement preparations available in the UK in the past five years with currently more than 50 available in different dose combinations. One survey, reported in 1998, estimated that 17 per cent of women received an HRT preparation, with most use in women aged 46–55 years, suggesting that the main indication for treatment remains symptom control (Hope *et al.* 1998). Compared with past surveys this suggested that British women's knowledge and use of HRT has increased. There is growing realisation that optimal skeletal benefit from HRT may demand long duration of use and this raises the necessity to consider approaches to HRT which would involve increased treatment and cost monitoring.

The RCT literature demonstrates that, if HRT is initiated at the onset of oestrogen deficiency, it will prevent expected bone loss in the majority of women for the duration of therapy. The extent to which bone density is maintained after cessation of therapy remains debatable but epidemiological data now suggest that a proportion of the skeletal benefit will be lost in later years if HRT is discontinued. Concern about breast cancer and other possible risks associated with extended HRT use and the awareness that bone loss may accelerate in old age have raised questions about the ideal times to initiate and discontinue therapy. In an attempt to address these questions, The Rancho Bernardo study (Schneider *et al.* 1997) has examined past and current use of HRT in a population based sample of more than 700 women. Their findings confirmed that continuous use of HRT from menopause into late life is associated with the highest bone density. However, HRT commenced after the age of 60 years appears to offer an almost equivalent effect (Figure 5.2). If late continuous use is equivalent to early onset continuous use, therapy could be started at older ages when most osteoporotic fractures occur, therefore reducing the cost and possible risks of long term HRT therapy.

Long term compliance with HRT and late onset of use are influenced by many actual and perceived variables and the continuing withdrawal bleed on sequential preparations has commonly been cited as the reason for discontinuing therapy. Data on the use of continuous combined therapies have revealed compliance rates of 80 per cent (Udoff *et al.* 1995) and it has been shown that three years use of continuous combined therapy had a significantly better effect on BMD than sequential therapy (Nielsen *et al.* 1994). The impact of continuous combined therapy on very long-term compliance remains unknown but its use may have major implications in the future.

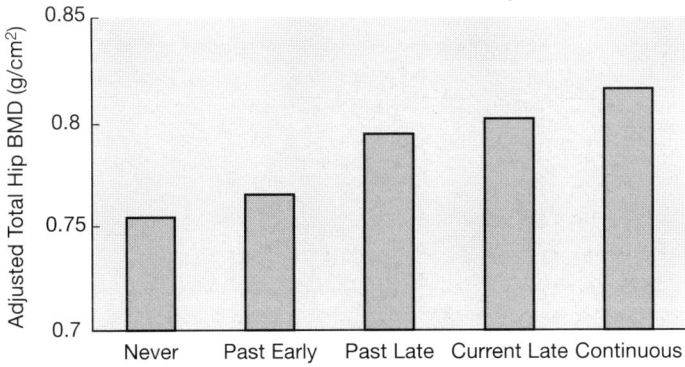

Figure 5.2 Adjusted bone mineral density at the total hip by oestrogen use groups. Data from Schneider *et al.* 1997.

Natural progesterone

The lay public is often tempted to use natural remedies as they are perceived to be risk free. It has been suggested by Lee that progesterone, not oestrogen deficiency, is the major cause of excess bone loss. His work demonstrated that the use of natural progesterone cream, derived from the wild yam, increased bone density by approximately 15 per cent (Lee 1991). Significant doubts have however been cast on the scientific reliability of these findings. A small study by Cooper (1997) suggested that the median plasma progesterone value achieved by the use of Progest cream was unlikely to have any biological effects on bone. Leonetti *et al.* showed that transdermal progesterone cream had no protective effect on bone density after one year (1999). Whilst this may appear another option for the prevention of osteoporosis, further research is required before it can be recommended.

Conclusion

In 1994, the Department of Health Advisory Group on Osteoporosis recognised the potential to improve existing approaches to the prevention and treatment of osteoporosis. In response to this, National Guidelines have recently been produced under the auspices of the Royal College of Physicians (1999). Evidence based methodology has been applied in the production of these guidelines and the recommendations of the document are systematically graded. Grade A recommendations are based on randomised controlled trials, whereas Grade B recommendations result from controlled studies without randomisation, studies with a quasi-experimental design and epidemiological studies. Grade C recommendations are based on expert committee reports or the clinical experience of recognised authorities.

The effect of lifestyle measures in the prevention of osteoporosis is shown in Table 5.1. Only exercise has been shown to improve bone density in randomised controlled trials (Grade A), but there is Grade B evidence that increasing dietary calcium intake and reducing tobacco consumption has a beneficial effect on bone density and the risk of vertebral and hip fractures. Pharmacological options for the prevention of osteoporosis include HRT at the time of ovarian failure (Grade A).

Observational data have identified many reversible factors, including low calcium intake and lack of physical activity that are associated with an increased risk of osteoporosis. Although more high quality evidence is required to show that decreasing the prevalence of these factors in the general population will increase bone mass, their reduction could lead to improvement in the public's health. Targeting prevention strategies at 'high risk' individuals represents an approach which may have greater impact on the prevention of osteoporosis. Another potentially avoidable risk factor is oestrogen deficiency, which can be corrected with HRT.

Reducing the incidence of osteoporosis through prevention will only become a reality if there is a combination of several strategies. Public health initiatives, for example, the inclusion of fall prevention strategies in Health Improvement

Table 5.1 The effect of lifestyle measures and HRT on bone density and the incidence of vertebral and hip fractures in the prevention of osteoporosis. Grading of recommendations adapted from Royal College of Physicians Clinical Guidelines for Prevention and Treatment of Osteoporosis (1999).

	Bone density	*Vertebral fractures*	*Hip fractures*
Exercise	A	B	B
Dietary calcium	B	B	B
↓ Smoking	B	B	B
↓ Alcohol	C	C	B
Oestrogen	A	B	B

Programmes represent one part of the picture. Accurate information about new aspects of diet, exercise and HRT from both health care professionals and the media will help individuals to make informed decisions about their health priorities. Although most of the responsibility will fall on the health services, educational initiatives could also be addressed through schools, the workplace and leisure outlets.

Ultimately, the success or failure of any prevention strategy will rest on the individual's perception of health, assessment of risk and willingness and ability to co-operate and adapt.

References

Alekel DC, Peterson C, St Germain A (1999). Isoflavone rich soy isolate exerts significant bone sparing in the lumbar spine of peri-menopausal women. *Journal of Bone and Mineral Research* **14**, S208.

Arjmandi BH, Alekel L, Hollis BW *et al.* (1996). Dietary soybean prevents bone loss in ovariectomised rat model of osteoporosis. *Journal of Nutrition* **126**, 161–167.

Berard A, Bravo G, Gauthier P (1997). Meta-analysis of the effectiveness of physical activity for the prevention of bone loss in *post-menopausal* women. *Osteoporosis International* **7**, 331–337.

Campbell JA, Robertson MC, Gardner MM, Norton RN, Tilyard MW, Buchner DM (1997). Randomised controlled trial of a general practice programme of home based exercise to prevent falls in elderly women. *British Medical Journal* **315**, 1065–1069.

Cooper A (1997). Absorption of progesterone from Progest cream. *Journal of the British Menopause Society* **3**, 23 (Advisory report).

Dawson-Hughes B, Harris SS, Krall EA, Dallal GE (1997). Effect of calcium and vitamin D supplementation on bone density in men and women 65 years of age or older. *New England Journal of Medicine* **337**, 670–676.

Gleeson PB, Protas E, LeBlanc A, Schneider VS, Evans HJ (1990). Effects of weight lifting on bone mineral density in *pre-menopausal* women. *Journal of Bone and Mineral Research* **5**, 153–158.

Ho SC, Chan SG, Wong EWM, Leung PC (1999). Soy intake and peak bone mass maintenance in Chinese women. *Journal of Bone and Mineral Research* **14**, S181.

Hope S, Wager E, Rees M (1998). Survey of British women's views on the menopause and HRT. *Journal of the British Menopause Society* **4**, 33–36.

Joakinsen RM, Magnus JH, Fonnebo J (1997). Physical activity and predisposition for hip fracture: a review. *Osteoporosis International* **7**, 503–513.

Johnell O, Gullberg B, Kanis JA, Allander AA, Elffors L, Dequeker J *et al.* (1995). Risk factors for hip fracture in European women: The MEDOS study. *Journal of Bone and Mineral Research* **10**, 1802–1815.

Kannus P, Haapasalo H, Sakelo M, Sievanen H, Pasanen M, Heinonen A *et al.* (1995). Effect of starting age of physical activity on bone mass in the dominant arm of tennis and squash players. *Annals of Internal Medicine* **123**, 27–31.

Krolner B, Toft B, Pars Nielsen S, Tondevold E (1983). Physical exercise as phrophylaxis against involutional bone loss: a controlled trial. *Clinical Science* **64**, 541–546.

Lanyon LE (1996). Using functional loading to influence bone mass and architecture: objectives, mechanisms, and relationship with estrogen of the mechanically adaptive process in bone. *Bone* **18**, S37–43.

Lee JR (1991). Is natural progesterone the missing link in osteoporosis prevention and treatment? *Medical Hypotheses* **36**, 178.

Leonetti HB, Longo S, Anasti JN (1999). Transdermal progesterone cream for vasomotor symptoms and *post-menopausal* bone loss. *Obstetrics and Gynaecology* **94**, 225–8.

Lloyd T, Andon MB, Rolloings N *et al.* (1993). Calcium supplementation and bone mineral density in adolescent girls. *Journal of the American Medical Association* **270**, 841–844.

Mackey R (1998). Phytoestrogens. *Journal of the British Menopause Society* **4**, 18–23.

Myers AH, Young Y, Langlois JA (1996). Prevention of falls in the elderly. *Bone* **18**, 87S–101S.

New SA, Bolton-Smith C, Grubb DA, Reid DM (1997). Nutritional influences on bone mineral density: a cross sectional study in *pre-menopausal* women. *American Journal of Clinical Nutrition* **65**, 1831–9.

Nielsen SP, Barenholdt O, Hermansen F, Munk-Jensen N (1994). Magnitude and pattern of skeletal response to long term continuous and cyclic sequential oestrogen/progestin treatment. *British Journal of Obstetrics and Gynaecology* **101**, 319–324.

Province MA, Hadley EC, Hornbrook MC *et al.* (1995). A preplanned meta-analysis of the FICSIT trials. *Journal of the American Medical Association* **273**, 1341–7.

Royal College of Physicians (1999). *Osteoporosis: Clinical Guidelines for Prevention and Treatment.* Royal College of Physicians, London.

Schneider DL, Barrett-Connor EL, Morton DJ (1997). Timing of *post-menopausal* estrogen for optimal bone mineral density. The Rancho Bernardo study. *Journal of the American Medical Association* **277**, 543–547.

Simkin A, Ayalon J, Leichter I (1987). Increased trabecular bone density due to bone loading exercises in *post-menopausal* women. *Calcified Tissue International* **40**, 503–513.

Slemenda C (1997). Prevention of hip fractures: risk factor modification. *American Journal of Medicine* **103**, 655–673.

Snow CM, Shaw JM, Matkin CC (1996). Physical activity and risk for osteoporosis. In: *Osteoporosis* (Marcus R, Feldman D, Kelsey J eds.). Academic Press, San Diego, pp511–28.

Tinetti ME, Speechley M, Ginter SF (1988). Risk factors for falls among elderly persons living in the community. *New England Journal of Medicine* **319**, 1701–7.

Tucker KL, Hannan MT, Chen H, Cupples AL, Wilson PWF, Kiel DP (1999). Potassium, magnesium, and fruit and vegetable intakes are associated with greater bone mineral density in elderly men and women. *American Journal of Clinical Nutrition* **69,** 727–36.

Udoff L, Langenberg P, Adashi EY (1995). Combined continuous hormone replacement therapy: a critical review. *Obstetrics and Gynaecology* **86,** 306–16.

Wachman A, Bernstein DS (1968). Diet and osteoporosis, *Lancet* **1**, 958–9.

Wolff I, Van Croonenborg JJ, Kemper HCG, Kostense PJ, Twisk JWR (1999). The effect of exercise training programs on bone mass: a meta-analysis of published controlled trials in pre and post-menopausal women. *Osteoporosis International* **9,** 1–12.

PART 3

Evidence and opinion in management and follow-up

Chapter 6

The role of calcium and vitamin D supplementation in complementing pharmacotherapy

Harpal Randeva and Gordana M Prelevic

Introduction

Bone is a dynamic tissue that is constantly remodelled throughout life. The rates of formation and resorption vary during the different stages of life but are particularly active while we are young. During growth, bone formation is relatively greater than bone resorption, in young adult life there is a balance between bone resorption and formation; and, usually after the third decade of life, there is an increase in bone resorption relative to bone formation. Bone does not only play a structural role for the organism but also acts as an internal reservoir for calcium and is an integral part of the calcium homeostatic system.

Calcium is the principal cation of bone mineral. An adult human contains approximately one kilogram of calcium (20–25g per kilograms lean body weight). Around 99 per cent of this calcium is in the skeleton in the form of hydroxyapatite, and 1 per cent is contained in the extracellular and intracellular fluids and soft tissues. About 1 per cent of the skeletal content of calcium appears to be freely exchangeable with extracellular fluid. It is this exchangeable pool which serves as an important buffer or storehouse of calcium. The extracellular concentration of calcium ions (Ca^{2+}) is in the range of 10–3 M, whereas the intracellular (cytosol) concentration of calcium is around 10–6 M. The low intracellular calcium level is maintained by calcium pumps and 90–99 per cent of intracellular calcium is bound to mitochondria and microsomes. Calcium is an important intracellular second messenger and is a cofactor for certain key intracellular enzymes. Likewise, extracellular calcium plays a crucial role for a variety of regulatory and metabolic activities such as serving as a cofactor in the coagulation cascade, excitation-contraction of the heart, normal functioning of muscle, nerves and haematological variables.

In the extracellular fluid, calcium circulates in three definable fractions: ionised or 'free' calcium (about 50 per cent) which is metabolically active and physiologically important, protein-bound calcium (about 40 per cent) and calcium that is complexed to anions such as bicarbonate, citrate and phosphate (about 10 per cent). Therefore approximately 60 per cent (both complex and ionised fraction) of the total calcium in serum is ultrafilterable. Approximately 90 per cent of the protein-bound calcium is associated with albumin, the remainder being complexed to globulin. Therefore any disorder that lowers serum albumin will lower total serum calcium concentration but have a lesser effect on ionised calcium concentration. It is extra cellular fluid pH which principally determines calcium binding to carboxyl groups in albumin. Acidosis will therefore decrease protein binding and increase ionised calcium, and alkalosis, through increase in binding will result in a consequent decrease in ionised calcium.

Apart from the physiological importance of ionised calcium described above, adequate concentrations of this divalent cation in extracellular fluid are required for normal rates of bone mineralisation. Systemic calcium homeostasis and maintenance of the normal serum calcium concentration in extracellular fluid, depends on integrated regulation of calcium fluxes across the gut, kidney, bone and other tissues.

The total extracellular pool of calcium is approximately 900 mg. In zero balance, bone resorption and formation are equivalent at about 500 mg per day. Calcium is both absorbed and secreted by the intestine, with a net absorption of approximately 175–200 mg per day. The filtered load of calcium in the kidney is 10g a day, with a net urinary excretion of only 175–200 mg of calcium, which balances the net intestinal absorption of calcium. The precise regulation of serum calcium is controlled by calcium itself, through a G-protein coupled calcium sensing receptor and several systemic hormones, most importantly parathyroid hormone (PTH) and 1,25-Dihydroxyvitamin $D_3(1,25(OH)_2D_3)$. The calcium sensing receptor responds to small, physiological changes in extracellular calcium and other divalent and trivalent cations, with transcripts of the receptor being identified in the parathyroid, kidney, thyroid C cells.

The parathyroid chief cells are exquisitely sensitive to changes in ionised serum calcium concentration. PTH has a direct action on the proximal and distal tubules of the kidneys, increases renal tubular reabsorption of calcium whilst decreasing reabsorption of phosphate. Parathyroid hormone also acts directly on the skeleton increasing the activity and number of osteoclasts and consequently bone resorption. These two direct effects of PTH are the major control points in minute-to-minute serum calcium homeostasis. A further important effect of PTH on the kidney is to stimulate the 1-alpha-hydroxylase enzyme responsible for the production of $1,25(OH)_2D_3$ from 25-Hydroxyvitamin $D_3(25-(OH)D_3)$; therefore, PTH indirectly acts on the intestine to normalise any fall in extracellular ionised calcium.

The principle effects of $1,25(OH)_2D_3$ on calcium metabolism are to enhance intestinal calcium absorption and phosphate by inducing the synthesis of several proteins. The main control of PTH secretion is determined by extracellular fluid ionised calcium although $1,25(OH)_2D_3$ suppresses PTH secretion directly as a short loop feedback. However, one cannot rely on PTH alone to maintain normal serum calcium if there is inadequate calcium intake in the diet. Longterm deficiency in dietary calcium will ultimately lead to a negative calcium balance, particularly from the bone, ultimately compromising the biochemical strength of bone.

Calcium availability for the skeleton is dependent not only on dietary intake, but also on intestinal absorption of calcium and renal tubular reabsorption of calcium. Apart from the physiological changes of ageing there are other physiological and pathological conditions that may affect calcium absorption and resorption.

Calcium absorption and resorption

In humans, only 25–35 per cent of dietary calcium is absorbed at contemporary intakes and a much smaller fraction at higher intakes. Although the amount of calcium absorbed is proportional to calcium intake, fractional absorption varies inversely with dietary intake, providing a partial compensation for dietary calcium insufficiency (Heaney *et al.* 1989). This adaptation results from the homeostatic regulation of 1,25-Dihydroxyvitamin D, the most potent modifier of calcium absorption. In addition, there are a number of systemic modulators of intestinal calcium absorption. Agents that increase calcium absorption include: PTH (through stimulation of synthesis of 1,25-Dihydroxyvitamin D), growth hormone, oestrogen therapy, pregnancy and lactation where there is an increased production of 1,25-Dihydroxyvitamin D, and frusemide which increases urinary calcium excretion with a compensatory increased intestinal calcium absorption. Phosphate depletion and a diet low in calcium and high in sodium, also increase calcium absorption.

Apart from ageing, which decreases intestinal calcium absorption, glucocorticoids, thyroid hormone and thiazide diuretics also reduce calcium absorption. Metabolic acidosis is also reported to reduce intestinal absorption of calcium as is a low sodium and a high calcium diet. A number of intraluminal factors affect intestinal calcium absorption. Phosphate, oxalate, dietary fibre and phytate reduce calcium absorption through the formation of insoluble complex long chain fatty acids. Tetracycline is known to bind calcium and therefore reduce calcium absorption as does small bowel resection. On the other hand certain amino acids such as lysine, arginine and certain antibiotics (penicillin, chloramphenicol) increase calcium absorption.

Similarly, regulation of urinary calcium excretion is dependent upon a number of dietary, hormonal and metabolic factors. A reduction in glomerular filtration rate will reduce urinary calcium excretion, whilst any factor which reduces renal tubular reabsorption will lead to increase in urinary calcium excretion. Increasing sodium in the diet and also increasing dietary protein intake is accompanied by increased urinary calcium excretion. On the other hand, phosphate administration leads to a fall in urinary calcium. The major effect of PTH, which occurs in the ascending loop of Henley and the distal tubule, is to enhance calcium reabsorption. Chronic glucocorticoid excess impairs renal calcium reabsorption. Likewise, chronic mineralocorticoid excess, insulin infusion and hyperinsulinaemia are associated with hypercalciuria. Diuretics such as frusemide and bumetanide inhibit tubular calcium reabsorption, whereas thiazide diuretics have the opposite effect leading to a decrease in urinary calcium excretion. Metabolic acidosis, both acute and chronic, is associated with an increase in calcium excretion.

Calcium requirements throughout lifetime

The age at which peak bone mass is achieved is at the end of the second decade (Matkovic *et al.* 1994; Teegarden *et al.* 1995), although it occurs at various times for different bones (Heaney 1995). Peak bone mass is determined by a combination of endogenous and exogenous factors (Ott 1991); although primarily under genetic control and mechanical loading, it cannot be achieved if calcium intake is insufficient. Furthermore, it should be emphasised that the rates of intestinal calcium absorption and renal calcium excretion, and excretory losses by the skin and bowel, vary with different stages of life and with other factors, as discussed above. Hence, calcium requirements vary at different stages of life.

The rate of bone modelling varies greatly through infancy, childhood and puberty. At birth the neonate has 25g of calcium. The skeletal mass (1000–1200 g) of infants doubles during the first year of life, with bone growth in adolescents accounting for 40–50 per cent of the total skeletal mass of adults (Bonjour *et al.* 1991). During adolescence calcium needs are greatest; adolescents absorb and retain more calcium from their diet (350 mg per day) than either children or young adults. Furthermore, net retention of calcium by the skeleton averages 100–150 mg per day for those up to the age of 11 and about 250 mg per day during adolescence. It is therefore important to note that if during adolescence the intake of calcium is very low (less than 500 mg per day), then adolescents, primarily because of greater obligatory loss of calcium in the urine, are in worse calcium balance than younger children.

Matkovic and Heaney (1992) were able to demonstrate the existence of an intake threshold for calcium in growing children. They observed that calcium intakes below a threshold value will produce more bone only up to the point at which the genetic potential is fully saturated and that intakes above the threshold level produced no further benefit. Needless to say, the exact threshold value depends on age and intakes of other nutrients. Therefore, during growth, calcium intakes lower than the threshold value are associated with lower retention of calcium by the skeleton and high intakes with greater retention.

During the adult years the cycle of bone remodelling (resorption and formation) continues, albeit at a slower rate. Although bone is no longer growing, obligatory losses of calcium (urine, faeces, skin and nails) make it essential that the calcium requirements in young adults are maintained to reach a positive calcium balance of 50 mg per day. During the later stages of life, particularly the menopause, calcium requirements are increased because of various factors. For example, there is an age related decrease in both intestinal absorption and renal tubular reabsorption of calcium, along with changes of several other hormones and growth factors, including oestrogens, androgens, growth hormone, insulin-like growth factor 1 and thyroid hormones, all of which regulate calcium homeostasis (Breslau 1996).

There is now a consensus view (NIH Consensus Conference 1994) regarding the intake of calcium that is optimal for growth and adult maintenance (Table 6.1). It is

Table 6.1 Optimal calcium requirements

Age	Daily calcium intake (mg)
Infants	
Birth–6 months	400
6 months–1 year	600
Children	
1–5 years	800
6–11 years	800–1200
Adolescents/adults	
12–24 years	1200–1500
Pregnancy/breast feeding	1200–1500
Men	
25–65 years	1000
> 65 years	1500
Women	
25–50 years	1000
> 50 years	1500

estimated to be 800–1000 mg per day during childhood, 1200–1500 mg per day from age 12–24 years, 1000 mg per day from age 25 to oestrogen deprivation and 1500 mg per day thereafter. The threshold values are above the recommended dietary allowances (RDAs). Calcium deficiency, particularly during skeletal formation, could decrease peak bone mass and thereby increase the risk of fracture later in life (Matkovic *et al.* 1977); this highlights the importance of optimising calcium requirements, principally through diet, e.g., dairy products, but also through calcium supplementation.

Calcium supplementation

The amount of calcium available for the skeleton and the body is dependent on the level of dietary intake, intestinal absorption efficiency and renal tubular reabsorption. It is clear from above that the intake 'threshold' for calcium varies with stages of life and the need for calcium being greatest during adolescence so that peak bone mass can be achieved. More importantly growing children and adolescents, unlike adults, need to be in a positive calcium balance. In children, calcium deficiency causes stunting and may also result in rickets (Kooh *et al.* 1977). Around 40–60 per cent of children's calcium intake comes from milk (Department of Health 1989).

Furthermore, a positive correlation between milk intake in childhood and at adolescence, and bone mineral density in post-menopausal women has been reported (Sandler *et al.* 1985; Murphy *et al.* 1994). It seems unlikely, given modern diet and culture, that the optimal calcium requirement for peak bone mass during adolescence could be acquired through dietary intake alone. Calcium supplementation could bridge the gap so that children and adolescents could ensure a positive calcium balance for bone growth and hence peak bone mass.

The need for calcium supplementation is also evident in adults. In a 14-year prospective study, the age-adjusted risk of hip fracture was inversely associated with dietary calcium intake; the risk persisted after adjustment for age, sex, body mass index, cigarette smoking and alcohol intake (Holbrook *et al.* 1988). During the adult years, even though bone modelling (shape changes) is not occurring, bone remodelling (material changes) together with increased excretion of calcium in the urine and faeces, and dermal losses, requires that young adults remain in a positive calcium balance of about 50 mg per day (Matkovic & Heaney 1992). Again in order to meet the recommended calcium requirements in young adults, in particular women of reproductive age, calcium supplementation may be needed in some.

It is clear that calcium intakes are positively correlated with bone mass at all ages, but in particular in post-menopausal women and in old age (Heaney *et al.* 1989). In the elderly, not only is there a decrease in dietary intake of calcium but intestinal absorption of calcium appears to fall whilst urinary excretion of calcium increases. This increased 'loss' of calcium must be drawn from the bone, consequently increasing calcium requirement. Recently it has been found that a defect in renal calcium conservation may contribute towards post-menopausal osteoporosis (Heshmati *et al.* 1998). In addition, low bone density has been shown to be an important predictor of future fracture risk (Cummings *et al.* 1990). The deficiency of calcium in elderly people, in particular those in sheltered accommodation, may partly explain the increased risk of hip fracture in this group. It is in this group that calcium supplementation is particularly important in order to meet optimal calcium requirements. The need for calcium supplementation, usually with vitamin D, is also recognised in patients who are on long term use of corticosteroids, which lead to loss of bone mineral density and increased risk of vertebral fractures (Warady *et al.* 1994). For these reasons, and for those who cannot or will not modify their diet in order to achieve their recommended intake of calcium, dietary supplements are often advised.

Calcium supplements are available in many forms (Table 6.2), including calcium gluconate, calcium lactate, calcium citrate, calcium carbonate and calcium phosphate. It should be noted that only elemental calcium is available for absorption, and the amount in each form of calcium supplement varies: calcium carbonate 40 per cent, calcium phosphate 39 per cent, calcium citrate 24 per cent, calcium lactate 13 per cent and calcium gluconate 9 per cent. However, the amount of calcium available for intestinal absorption, in other words calcium bioavailability, may vary amongst

Table 6.2 Calcium preparations

Salt	Preparation	mg of Ca^{2+}/tab
Gluconate	calcium gluconate	54
	effervescent calcium gluconate	90
Carbonate	calcium-500	500
	calcichew	500
	citrical	500
	calcidrink	1000
Citrate	cacit	500
Lactate	calcium lactate	40
Hydroxyapatite	ossopan	176
		712
Lactonate gluconate, carbonate	sandocal	400
		1000

these preparations because of the low aqueous solubility of certain preparations (carbonate and phosphate) and also the ability of some salts (citrate) to form soluble complexes with calcium (Pak *et al.* 1986). Another important factor which may affect bioavailability is the pH of gastric juice. In the elderly and in patients following treatment with antacids or H$_2$ blockers and those with achlorhydria, calcium bioavailability from carbonate and phosphate salts is low because of their incomplete dissolution (Recker 1985). Likewise, anions released from lactate, citrate and carbonate salts may neutralise part of the gastric acid and impair solubility of calcium salts. With these factors in mind, and studies comparing calcium bioavailability from calcium citrate to that of calcium carbonate (Nicar & Pak 1985; Pak *et al.* 1986), it is believed that calcium citrate may provide optimum calcium bioavailability. However, the most widely used calcium supplement remains calcium carbonate.

The dose of calcium supplement varies with different age groups. However, it is clear from Table 6.1 that the 'optimal' calcium requirement is more than the current recommended daily allowance. The absorption of calcium and hence bioavailability, is affected by factors such as dose and timing of supplements and concurrent medications. It is known that the fractional absorption of calcium varies inversely with calcium intake (Heaney *et al.* 1989). In addition, absorption is complete within four hours of calcium intake and is more efficient at low intakes of calcium. Therefore, given that intestinal calcium absorption is a saturable and energy dependent transport process, and that the percentage of calcium absorbed is more when a fixed amount of calcium is taken in divided doses as compared to a single dose, calcium supplements should be prescribed 3–4 times daily (Heaney 1991). Furthermore, intestinal calcium absorption is improved if supplements are taken with meals. It is known that bone turnover shows a circadian rhythm, being most active during the night. Therefore, evening/night time calcium supplementation seems to be the most effective (Blumsohn *et al.* 1994).

The effect of dietary calcium intake on bone mineral density and fracture

Peak bone mass, which occurs towards the late 20s is mainly under the influence of genetic factors. However, there is evidence that it can be enhanced by increased calcium intake (Matkovic *et al.* 1990). This effect of calcium is seen throughout life, but particularly during adolescence when the need for calcium is higher in order to maintain a 'positive' balance so that the extra skeletal requirements can be met. It is known that low calcium intakes in childhood are associated not only with an increased risk of osteoporosis later in life, but with an increased fracture risk in adolescence (Chan *et al.* 1994; Heaney 1996). The importance of calcium on skeletal growth was evident in a study conducted by Orr (1928), who showed that children who drank milk were taller than their peers who did not. In a prospective study, where calcium intake was recorded every six months from birth to five years, Lee *et al.* (1993) were able to demonstrate a positive correlation between longterm calcium intake and bone mineral density at the wrist.

In adolescence there is a need for positive calcium balance, and the higher the calcium intake the greater the calcium retention, with the maximal retention occurring just after menarche (Jackman *et al.* 1997). Interestingly, a high calcium intake during adolescence and young adulthood, has been shown to be positively associated with greater peak bone mass and bone mineral density in adult life (Sandler *et al.* 1985; Bauer *et al.* 1993; Murphy *et al.* 1994). In a community-based cross sectional study, Murphy *et al.* (1994) were able to show that frequent milk consumption before the age of 25 was a significant independent predictor of bone mineral density in middle aged and older women. Likewise, in a three-year study, an additional 600 mg per day in calcium intake, provided in the form of dairy products, was reported to result in less bone loss, with beneficial effects on spine bone mineral density, as compared to the placebo group (Baran *et al.* 1990). Furthermore, a meta-analysis of calcium intake and bone mass has found that calcium has more of an impact on cortical bone rather than cancellous bone, i.e., hip versus spine bone mineral density (Cumming 1990).

Only a few studies have looked at the relationship between calcium intake and hip fracture, and these have produced conflicting results. In a 14-year longitudinal study, Holbrook *et al.* (1988) were able to demonstrate a protective and anti-fracture effect of calcium, as individuals on high calcium intake were observed to have fewer fractures. However, there are a number of prospective studies, looking at the role of calcium in fracture risk, which have not found any protection between calcium intake and fracture risk (Wickham *et al.* 1989; Paganini-Hill *et al.* 1991; Cummings *et al.* 1995). These conflicting findings may have arisen due to a number of factors: different ranges of dietary calcium, defects in the design of the study, unstandardised dietary assessments. A study by Matkovic *et al.* (1979), comparing fracture rates in two regions of Yugoslavia, found a 60–75 per cent lower incidence of hip fractures in women in the region where dietary calcium was around 1,000 mg a day, compared to the other region where women ingested half that intake. Similar observations have been reported by others (Holbrook *et al.* 1988; Recker *et al.* 1996). Likewise, the risk of hip fractures was significantly lower in women in the highest quartile of calcium intake as compared with the lowest quartile, but this observation was only noted in the subgroup of women who were at least six years post-menopausal (Looker *et al.* 1993). On balance, the relationship between calcium intake and fracture risk in post-menopausal women is suggestive of a beneficial effect.

The effect of calcium supplementation on bone mineral density and fracture

The beneficial effects of calcium supplementation in seven-year-old children accustomed to a low calcium diet, were shown in a double blind controlled study by Lee *et al.* (1994). However, the same authors showed that the benefits of calcium were only evident while calcium supplements were taken, as bone mineral density returned to that of the controlled group in their follow-up study (Lee *et al.* 1996). In another three-year double-blind placebo controlled trial in pre-pubertal (10–12 years) monozygotic twins (Johnston *et al.* 1992), in whom the dietary intake of calcium approximated the recommended dietary allowance (RDA), calcium supplementation (700 mg per day) increased their bone mineral density faster than the controls (monozygotic twins). However, like the study by Lee *et al.* (1996) the effects on bone mineral density were lost when supplementation was discontinued, suggesting the importance of maintaining calcium intake throughout adolescence and adulthood (Slemends *et al.* 1993). Similar findings of the beneficial effects of calcium supplementation in both pre- and post-pubertal healthy children have been shown in other randomised trials (Lloyd *et al.* 1993; Cadogan *et al.* 1997). The above studies suggest that peak bone mass can be optimised by supplementing the diet with calcium even in those children and adolescents considered to be taking an 'adequate' intake of calcium.

The effect of calcium supplementation in pre-menopausal women has been a subject of debate. In a four-year study of calcium supplementation (500 mg a day) in middle aged women, Smith *et al.* (1989) found no significant effect on bone mineral density. Other studies have shown otherwise. In a longitudinal study, in eugonadal women, where 1,000 mg of calcium supplementation were given each day, there was significant increase in total body bone mineral density after one year (Rico *et al.* 1995). In another longitudinal study, by Recker *et al.* (1992), involving nearly 200 healthy women in their 20s, the investigators were able to demonstrate that additional calcium supplementation beyond the recommended daily allowance (RDA) augmented bone gain, a finding also observed by Matkovic & Heaney (1992). These findings have also been confirmed in children (Lee *et al.* 1993). Furthermore, the study by Recker *et al.* (1992) found that the rate of bone gain was inversely proportional to age and that the principal determinant of the amount of bone gain was the calcium to protein ratio of diet. It would therefore seem that calcium supplementation in healthy women of reproductive age has a protective action against bone loss.

The value of calcium supplementation on the rate of bone loss after the menopause, has been the subject of considerable debate. However, the general consensus is that calcium supplementation reduces the rate of age-related bone loss (Dawson-Hughes 1991). A review of 20 respective trials in post-menopausal women given calcium supplementations, concluded that there was a reduction in bone loss of about 1 per cent per year (Nordin 1997). The conflicting data on the relationship between calcium supplementation and bone mass in post-menopausal women, may in part be related to a number of factors, such as intrinsic errors in dietary histories, the site of the skeleton used to determine bone density, the dose and type of calcium supplementation and, more importantly, the timing of the study in relation to the menopause.

In a randomised trial by Elders *et al.* (1994), comparing the bone mineral density of older pre-menopausal women and early post-menopausal women given calcium supplementation (1,000–2,000 mg of calcium), it was found that calcium supplementation significantly reduced spinal bone density loss in the pre-menopausal but not in the post-menopausal women. Other trials have also failed to show the beneficial effect of calcium supplementation on bone mineral density during the first five years after the menopause (Dawson-Hughes *et al.* 1990; Reid & New 1997). The study by Dawson-Hughes *et al.* (1990), found that among women with low basal calcium intake (400 mg per day or less) calcium supplementation was more effective in late post-menopausal women (six or more years since the menopause). This beneficial effect of calcium supplementation (1,000 mg per day) on bone mineral density in late menopausal woman has been confirmed by Reid *et al.* (1993). Furthermore, in the same study, in which calcium intake was increased from 750 mg to 1,750 mg per day, Reid *et al.* were able to demonstrate the intake level of calcium at which a skeletal benefit is observed in women several years after the menopause. Similarly, the work by Lau *et al.* (1992) revealed that a low calcium intake leads to bone loss in elderly women, but increasing the calcium intake from 800 to 1,000 mg daily by supplementation reduces this loss. All these studies highlight the importance of calcium supplementation in reducing bone loss in late post-menopausal women. Therefore, early in the menopausal period, bone loss may be primarily regarded as a consequence of gonadal hormone deficiency and in the later menopausal years it is predominantly due to calcium deficiency. Furthermore, the elevated biomarkers for bone resorption and high circulating parathyroid hormone levels, typical of the elderly, are reversible with a higher calcium intake (McKane *et al.* 1996). Therefore, calcium can be regarded as a threshold nutrient, the threshold value depending on other nutrients and physiological state (e.g., oestrogen deficiency) and the threshold value may differ by skeletal site.

The benefits of calcium supplementation are seen more in appendicular cortical bone, with a less prominent and transient effect on the axial skeleton, the site at which two of the most important osteoporotic fractures occur, that is the spine and the hip. Studies by Elders *et al.* (1994) and Aloia *et al.* (1994), have shown a positive effect of calcium supplementation on lumbar spine bone mass; however, this effect was not maintained after one year of calcium supplementation. In the same study by Aloia *et al.*, significant beneficial effects of calcium supplementation on bone mineral density at the femoral neck were noted, but not in Ward's Triangle, a finding also reported by Dawson-Hughes *et al.* (1990). However, in the study by Reid *et al.* (1993) in post-menopausal women, the findings were converse, with beneficial effects of calcium on bone mass at Ward's Triangle but not the femoral neck.

Calcium supplementation has also been linked to reduced fracture rates in post-menopausal women. In a prospective, double-blind study, Chevalley *et al.* (1994) noted a significant reduction in vertebral fracture rate in vitamin D replete elderly subjects given 800 mg of calcium daily. Recker *et al.* (1996) demonstrated that supplemental calcium (1,200 mg a day) significantly reduced the incidence of vertebral fractures in women with low calcium intakes (mean 433 md/day). In a large case control study of over 5,000 population-based women, of whom just over 2,000 had sustained a hip fracture, calcium supplementation was associated with a significant reduction in the relative risk of fracture, by approximately 30 per cent (Kanis *et al.* 1992). The benefits of long term calcium supplementation on reduction of fracture risk, have also been shown by Reid *et al.* (1995).

Vitamin D

Vitamin D is a secosteroid with diverse biological actions. It is essential for skeletal health, maintaining calcium homeostasis via its action at the level of intestine and bone. Vitamin D is rare in foods, with only about 10 per cent being derived from the diet. Ergocalciferol (vitamin D_2) is a form of vitamin D found in plants and yeast and cholecalciferol (vitamin D_3) is the form found in fatty fish, fish liver oils and other animal sources. Both compounds have equivalent biological activity in humans. These dietary forms of vitamin D are fat soluble substances which are primarily absorbed from the proximal small bowel, where, on incorporation into chylomicron, a fraction are absorbed and transported through the lymphatic system. Vitamin D has a half-life of approximately 48 hours and is stored in fat and muscles. In individuals with fat malabsorption disorders (e.g., Coeliac disease, pancreatic insufficiency) absorption of vitamin D may fail.

The skin is the major source of vitamin D. Exposure to ultraviolet B radiation, with a spectrum of 290–315 nm, leads to the conversion of 7-dehydrocholesterol (7-DHC, pro-vitamin D_3), the immediate precursor of cholesterol, to pre-vitamin D_3 (Holick 1995b). This product is thermodynamically unstable and hence isomerizes to vitamin D_3 over a period of a few hours. Vitamin D_3 is then translocated form the epidermis into the circulation by the vitamin D binding protein (VDBP). There are mechanisms in place which prevent vitamin D intoxication after prolonged UV light exposure, namely the conversion of pre-vitamin D_3 to inert photo products, lumisterol and tachysterol, and likewise vitamin D_3 is converted to suprasterol 1 and 2 and 5,6-trans-vitamin D_3. Hence with protector mechanisms in place only about 15 per cent of total cutaneous 7-DHC is converted to pre-vitamin D_3, irrelevant to the length of UV light exposure (Holick 1995b).

The cutaneous production of vitamin D_3 may be influenced by a variety of factors such as ageing, melanin, sunscreens, latitude, season and time of day. Ageing significantly diminishes the concentration of 7-DHC in the epidermis, which consequently leads to a reduction in the production of vitamin D_3, by up to 30 per cent less as compared to a young adult (Holick et $al.$ 1989). Sunscreens with a sun protection factor of 8 will substantially reduce (greater than 95 per cent) the cutaneous production of vitamin D_3 (Holick 1995b). Melanin, an excellent natural sunscreen produced by the body, competes with 7-DHC for ultraviolet B radiation which in turn leads to a decreased production pre-vitamin D_3 in the skin. The capacity to produce vitamin D_3 in the skin is the same irrespective of skin colour; however, compared to those with lighter skin colour, people with darker skin colour require longer exposure time to sunlight to make the same amount of vitamin D_3 (Holick 1994).

At a latitude of 42 degrees north (e.g., Boston, USA), the skin is incapable of producing vitamin D_3 between the months of November and February. At 55 degrees north (e.g., Glasgow, UK) this period is extended to include the months of October to April. In Boston during the summer months, exposure during the hours of 0700 to 1700 contains sufficient ultraviolet radiation to produce vitamin D_3 but in the autumn and spring, production commences at 0900 hours and ceases at 1500 hours.

Despite the various factors that may influence cutaneous production of vitamin D_3, it remains biologically inert and, like dietary sources of vitamin D, it must undergo successive hydroxylation in the liver and kidney to become biologically active. Once vitamin D enters the circulation from the skin or diet, it is bound to the vitamin D binding protein and transported to the liver where it is metabolised to the major circulating form of vitamin D, 25-Hydroxyvitamin D (25-OHD).

Metabolism of vitamin D

In the liver the vitamin D-25-hydroxylase enzyme metabolises vitamin D to 25-OHD, the principal form of vitamin D in circulation. It is produced in a relatively unregulated fashion, i.e., the hepatic vitamin D-25-hydroxylase enzyme is not tightly regulated. Consequently, increased production of vitamin D (cutaneous or ingestion) will lead to increased circulating levels of 25-OHD. Hence, the serum concentration of 25-OHD is the best clinical measure of vitamin D status. There are a number of factors that may influence 25-OHD concentrations: severe cholestatic or hepatocellular disease (Long *et al.* 1976), anti-convulsant therapy (Phenytoin, Phenobarbitone) which increases the catabolism of 25-OHD and the nephrotic syndrome where there is loss in the urine of VDBP with its tightly bound 25-OHD (Pietrek & Kokot 1977). In addition, sarcoidosis, obesity, primary and secondary hyperparathyroidism and vitamin D dependent rickets type II (Bell 1985), increase the metabolism of 25-OHD.

Although 25-OHD is two to five times more active than vitamin D, at physiological concentrations it is biologically inert. In the kidney, 25-OHD undergoes further hydroxylation under the influence of 1-alpha-hydroxylase enzyme to form $1,25(OH)_2D$, the hormonally active metabolite of vitamin D (Holick 1995b). In contrast to 25-hydroxylation in the liver, 1-alpha-hydroxylation is under exquisite metabolic control through factors that influence the renal 1-alpha-hydroxylase enzyme. Factors which stimulate this enzyme are PTH, hypocalcaemia, growth hormone, prolactin, hypophosphataemia and sex steroids. The enzyme is inhibited by hypercalcaemia, hyperphosphataemia and high concentrations of $1,25(OH)_2D$. In certain situations, which will not be covered in this chapter, 25-OHD may also be converted to the inactive 24,25-Dihydroxyvitamin D.

Apart from the kidney, which is the major source of circulating $1,25(OH)_2D$, a wide variety of other cells including bone and skin cells have the ability to produce $1,25(OH)_2D$ as does the placenta. $1,25(OH)_2D$ has a half-life of six hours and is metabolised in target tissues such as intestine, bone, liver and kidneys. It is approximately ten times more active than 25-OHD and is responsible for the physiological actions of 'vitamin D'.

Actions of vitamin D

The mechanism of action of vitamin D is similar to that of other steroids. All target tissues for vitamin D contain a specific, high affinity nuclear vitamin D receptor (VDR) which has 1,000 fold higher affinity for $1,25(OH)_2D$ compared to 25-OHD. The VDR is not only found in 'calcaemic tissues' (small bowel, bone and kidneys) but VDR activity is also seen in non-calcaemic tissues e.g., pituitary, gonads, prostate, breast and others (Holick 1995a). The VDR along with $1,25(OH)_2D$ and the retinoic acid X receptor (RXR), form a heterodimer complex which interacts with the vitamin D responsive element (VDRE) leading to the transcription of the gene and synthesis of mRNAs for a variety of proteins. These proteins are in turn responsible for the major biological functions of vitamin D, namely calcium homeostasis, bone metabolism and other actions on non-calcaemic tissues such as the immune system and the regulation of cell proliferation and differentiation.

Vitamin D [1,25(OH)$_2$D] maintains calcium homeostasis by a number of mechanisms. It increases the efficiency of the small intestine to absorb dietary calcium and phosphorus through its VDRs. 1,25(OH)$_2$D increases the concentration of several proteins in the small intestine such as alkaline phosphatase, calcium binding proteins, calcium ATPase, and calmodulin, although the exact mechanism by which vitamin D alters the flux of calcium across the intestinal cell is not known. Vitamin D also maintains calcium homeostasis through its action on bone by inducing stem cells in the bone to differentiate into osteoclasts (Holick 1995b), at times when dietary calcium intake is low. However, osteoclasts do not express the VDR and therefore osteoclastic-mediated bone resorption appears to be regulated indirectly by 1,25(OH)$_2$D through its action on VDRs on osteoblasts; the latter produce a variety of osteoclast-sensitive cytokines and hormones. In addition, 1,25(OH)$_2$D promotes the mineralisation of osteoid, laid down by osteoblasts, by maintaining extra cellular calcium homeostasis. In addition to its effects on calcium homeostasis and bone metabolism, 1,25(OH)$_2$D acts on the parathyroid gland to decrease PTH formation, and on kidneys it decreases its own synthesis and synergises with PTH to stimulate renal tubular reabsorption of calcium.

Consequences of vitamin D deficiency

Vitamin D has an important role in the mineralisation of the skeleton at all ages. As stores of vitamin D deplete, intestinal calcium absorption decreases, which leads to a fall in ionised calcium concentrations, and consequently to an increase in the synthesis and secretion of PTH (secondary hyperparathyroidism). PTH attempts to increase serum calcium by increasing renal tubular calcium reabsorption (and excretion of phosphorus), stimulating 1,25(OH)$_2$D synthesis which activate monocytic stem cells to become active calcium resorbing osteoclasts. The net effect is a normal/low serum calcium and phosphorus, elevated PTH and alkaline phosphatase. The level of 1,25(OH)$_2$D depends on the degree of 25-OHD deficiency and may be maintained in the normal range through the stimulation of the 1-alpha-hydroxylase enzyme by PTH. The consequences of a lack of vitamin D on bone will depend on the plasma concentrations of 25-OHD.

Hypovitaminosis D could be defined as a value of serum 25-OHD below which there is a risk for abnormalities to occur, i.e., a risk threshold. The cut-off levels, based on earlier findings (Parfitt *et al.* 1982), have approximated between 25–30 nmol/L. However, since then, based on a relationship between 25-OHD and PTH status, various authors have suggested threshold levels between 80 and 110 nmol/L (Heaney 1986; Dawson-Hughes *et al.* 1997; McKenna *et al.* 1997). In addition, terms such as vitamin D insufficiency and deficiency, which have been used synonymously, have again had different threshold levels to define them. The discrepancies between various publications may partly be due to different reference ranges of the 25-OHD assays. Vitamin D insufficiency, where biochemical tests such as 1,25(OH)$_2$D and

PTH may be borderline and improve following vitamin D supplementation, could be defined as a threshold level of serum 25-OHD between 25 and 50 nmol/L. The term vitamin D deficiency, in keeping with recommendation (Parfitt *et al.* 1982), describes an individual who has a definite abnormality that is reversible with a vitamin D supplementation and where serum 25-OHD levels are below 25 nmol/L. In this group PTH is raised with lowered 1,25(OH)$_2$D, with clinical features of vitamin D deficiency. Therefore, in general, hypovitaminosis D, vitamin D insufficiency and vitamin D deficiency could be defined by a serum 25-OHD level of less than 100 nmol/L, between 25 and 50 nmol/L and less than 25 nmol/L, respectively (McKenna & Freaney 1998).

Skeletal consequences of a lack of 25-OHD depend on its serum levels. Vitamin D deficiency will prevent sufficient amounts of 1,25(OH)$_2$D being produced, despite the increase in PTH. In combination with a low serum calcium and phosphate there is a delay in the rate of mineralisation of osteoid as it is laid down osteoblast, leading to a reduction in mineralised bone and reduced bone strength. The clinical picture is one of rickets in children and osteomalacia in adults. The soft elastic bone in osteomalacia deforms easily leading to scoliosis, kyphosis and deformities of the pelvis, rib cage and long bones. Vitamin D insufficiency also causes a reduced calcium supply and secondary hyperparathyroidism, albeit of a milder degree than found in vitamin D deficiency. The secondary hyperparathyroidism results in increased bone turnover and bone loss, leading to osteopaenia or osteoporosis. This state of vitamin D insufficiency is most commonly found in the elderly, where a PTH-mediated increase in bone turnover contributes to bone loss in both non-fracture (Compston 1995) and fracture (Aaron *et al.* 1974) patients. Certainly a mixture of both osteoporosis and osteomalacia (osteoporomalacia) may occur, particularly in the elderly.

Recommended intakes of vitamin D

On the whole, the requirement for vitamin D is satisfied by endogenous synthesis. It is clear that requirements for vitamin D vary according to a number of factors including age, seasonal variation in cutaneous exposure to UV light and other factors as described earlier. In general, for adults this is 200 IU per day. Individuals of certain countries, such as North America and Scandinavia, where food is fortified with vitamin D, have better vitamin D status in comparison to individuals from western and central Europe (McKenna 1992). The recommended daily allowance (RDA) of vitamin D for different age groups is shown in Table 6.3.

In 1997, the National Academy of Sciences and the Institute of Medicine in the United States reviewed the RDA of vitamin D. Based on observed and experimentally determined approximations of vitamin D intake by a defined population, their committee recommended an adequate intake (AI) of vitamin D for the various age groups, as shown in Table 6.3. The committee was quick to recognise that, in infants and individuals up to the age of 18 years and those who were pregnant or lactating, the

Table 6.3 Recommended dietary allowance (RDA) and adequate intake (AI) for Vitamin D.

Age	RDA IU/day	AI IU/day
0–6 months	300	200
6 months–12 yr	300	200
1–18 yr	400	200
19–50 yr	200	200
51–70 yr	200	400
> 71 yr	200	600
Pregnancy & lactation	400	200

adequate intakes were lower than previous recommended dietary allowances. They also appreciated that individuals who live in far northern and southern latitudes required higher dietary vitamin D levels in order to maintain maximum skeletal health, and that in these individuals 400 IU per day was considered not to be excessive. Adults aged between 19 and 50 years of age obtain most of their vitamin D requirement from cutaneous exposure to sunlight. However, in a study involving young adult male submariners, who were not exposed to any sunlight, it was noted that they required 600 IU per day of vitamin D in order to maintain normal serum 25-OHD levels (Holick 1994). Hence, an AI of 200 IU/day was recommended for this age group, regardless of exposure to sunlight.

In those aged over 51 years there is decreased cutaneous production of vitamin D, decreased outdoor activity and poor diet, all culminating in vitamin insufficiency/deficiency. In a study of over 300 ambulatory Caucasian women living in Boston, USA, Krall *et al.* (1989) reported no seasonal variation in PTH concentration when vitamin D intakes were greater than 220 IU per day. In addition, rates of bone loss in the spine were less in women assigned 400 IU per day of vitamin D compared to those given 200 IU per day (Dawson-Hughes *et al.* 1995). Similarly, men and women over 70 years of age require between 400–800 IU of vitamin D per day in order to maintain normal serum 25-OHD and PTH levels (Lips *et al.* 1988; Dawson-Hughes *et al.* 1995), and in order to increase bone mineral content (Dawson-Hughes *et al.* 1997). A study by Thomas *et al.* in 1998 found that of 290 patients on a general medical ward, 57 per cent had vitamin D insufficiency (less than 37.5 nmol/L) and 22 per cent had vitamin D deficiency (less than 20 nmol/L). This data would suggest that the current recommended adequate intakes of vitamin D are inadequate.

Finally, excessive ingestion of vitamin D can cause hypervitaminosis D. It is therefore recommended that the upper threshold safe intake level for those up to one year of age is 1,000 IU per day, and those over one year 2,000 IU per day.

Supplementation with vitamin D and its metabolites

There are a variety of physiological and pathological conditions where diet alone is unable to maintain normal vitamin D levels, necessitating vitamin D supplementation. One of the most important physiological causes of vitamin D deficiency is advancing age. A number of factors contribute to vitamin D deficiency in the elderly, namely low dietary intake of the vitamin, poor absorption, reduced sunlight exposure with impaired cutaneous synthesis of vitamin D, reduced hepatic and renal synthesis of 25-OHD and $1,25(OH)_2D$, respectively (Holick 1994). Elderly individuals who are housebound or institutionalised, are at a greater risk of developing osteomalacia and osteopaenia. It is in these individuals that the need for vitamin D supplementation is even more important.

A combination of increased skin pigmentation and reduced sunlight exposure (strict dress codes), exposes immigrants, in particular Asians, to the risk of developing vitamin D insufficiency/deficiency. Hence, most brands of chappati flour are fortified with vitamin D. Another group of individuals who are at risk of vitamin D insufficiency are vegans. Individuals with fat malabsorption syndromes such as Crohn's disease, tropical sprue, Whipples disease, and those with hepatobiliary disorders, or those who have undergone gastric surgery, are at risk of osteomalacia and osteopaenia. Apart from these individuals the need for vitamin D supplementation should also be borne in mind for those on anti-convulsant therapy (Phenytoin, Phenobarbitone), individuals taking Rifampicin and in those with nephrotic syndrome. Finally, insufficiency of the active vitamin D metabolite $[1,25(OH)_2D]$ can be seen in patients' chronic renal failure.

A number of preparations of vitamin D and its metabolites (e.g., alfacalcidol and calcitriol) are available. However, there is uncertainty as to the best dose and route of administration. Vitamin D can be given as an oral dose of 50,000 IU twice a week (Holick 1995b), or can even be given in a single oral dose of 100,000 IU once weekly, reducing problems associated with poor compliance. Alternatively, vitamin D can be given orally in regular daily doses of 400–800 IU, ensuring 25-OHD levels in the normal range and a reduction of serum PTH concentrations (Lips *et al.* 1988). It can also be given parenterally, either as a single intramuscular injection of 300,000 units every six months or as a single dose of 600,000 units every 6–12 months (Burns & Paterson 1985). The parenteral route is particularly useful in those with vitamin D deficiency associated with malabsorption.

Vitamin D metabolites can also be used and are particularly useful in patients with vitamin D deficiency associated with severe liver dysfunction, or in states where there is a defect in metabolism of 25-OHD to $1,25(OH)_2D$, for example, in patients with chronic renal failure and hypoparathyroidism. The daily dose of calcitriol is about one half of that for alfacalcidol.

Effect of vitamin D and its metabolites on bone mineral density and fracture risk

The importance of vitamin D and its implications on bone status, come from studies relating vitamin D intake/levels to PTH concentrations, bone mineral density, rates of bone loss, along with intervention studies looking at the effect of vitamin D on bone density and fracture rates.

Serum PTH is inversely correlated with serum 25-OHD (Thomas *et al.* 1988). Secondary hyperparathyroidism increases bone turnover and contributes to bone loss (Aaron *et al.* 1974). Not only does vitamin D supplementation lead to an increase in serum vitamin D values and intestinal calcium absorption, but it leads to a concomitant decrease of serum PTH, without simultaneous changes in serum calcium (Chapuy *et al.* 1987; Lips *et al.* 1988). In addition, vitamin D substitution is associated with a significant decrease in bone turnover rate (Prestwood *et al.* 1996). The observation of a seasonal variation in bone mineral density can be explained by the changes in 25-OHD and PTH levels. During the winter months there is marked loss of bone mineral density (hip and spine), related to a decrease in the cutaneous instances of 25-OHD and secondary hyperparathyroidism. During the summer, the reverse is true where serum 25-OHD levels increase and are associated with a reciprocal change in PTH and bone mineral density (Dawson-Hughes *et al.* 1991).

There are a number of studies demonstrating a correlation between bone density and serum 25-OHD concentrations (Dawson-Hughes *et al.* 1991; Khaw *et al.* 1992), where vitamin D insufficiency has been attributed to bone loss in perimenopausal women (Lukert *et al.* 1992). Supplementation of vitamin D in women in pre- and early- post-menopausal stage, has shown a beneficial effect on the skeleton. In studies comparing bone mineral density in women ingesting either 200 IU per day or 400 IU per day, investigators were able to demonstrate that those receiving the higher dose of vitamin D had less bone loss in the spine (Dawson-Hughes *et al.* 1991, 1995). There are a number of intervention studies supporting the need for vitamin D supplementation.

In a prospective, randomised study in 3,270 elderly women, with a mean calcium intake of 500 mg per day, Chapuy *et al.* (1992) observed that supplementation with 800 IU per day of cholecalciferol plus elemental calcium 1.2 g per day, increased femoral bone density by 2.7 per cent, compared to a decline of 4.6 per cent in placebo recipients. In another randomised, controlled trial in 249 healthy, post-menopausal women, daily supplementation with vitamin D (400 IU), given for one year, increased bone density of the spine (Dawson-Hughes *et al.* 1991). More recently, other randomised trials have also reported beneficial effects on bone mineral density. The study by Ooms *et al.* in 1995 in which 348 post-menopausal women were given 400 IU cholecalciferol daily for two years, showed that those receiving supplementation had an increased bone density at the femoral neck as compared to the placebo group. In another trial, men and women over the age of 65 years were randomised to treatment with placebo or 500 mg of elemental calcium plus 700 IU of vitamin D daily. Over a three-year period, supplementation significantly increased bone density at the femoral neck, spine and total body, as compared to placebo recipients (Dawson-Hughes *et al.* 1997)

The use and effectiveness of vitamin D metabolites are controversial. In the early post-menopause, both alfacalcidol and calcitriol showed no effect on bone mineral density (Christiansen *et al.* 1980, 1981). However, controlled trials conducted with these analogues in patients with osteoporosis provide some beneficial effects on bone mineral density. Again the data is controversial: no beneficial effect has been noted in studies from Northern Europe (Christiansen *et al.* 1980, 1981) although positive effects have been reported from Japan and elsewhere (Fujita 1990; Tilyard *et al.* 1992; Sambrook *et al.* 1993; Menczel *et al.* 1995). It should be noted that the significant and beneficial effects on bone mineral density were at the lumbar spine and not the femoral neck. The discrepancies seen in these studies, like others discussed below, may be related to a number of factors. In particular, dietary calcium intake may play an important part, as it is possible that the positive effects on bone mineral density are due to the increased absorption of calcium and not to a specific direct action of the vitamin D metabolite on bone.

Over the last decade a number of randomised controlled trials have addressed the effects of vitamin D supplementation on fracture rate. In the study by Chapuy *et al.* (1992), as described above, the mean age of the women was 84 years and they were living in residential nursing homes. After completion of the eighteen month study, of vitamin D (800 IU/day) and calcium (1.2 g/day) supplementation, the number of hip fractures was 43 per cent lower and the total number of non-vertebral fractures was 32 per cent lower among women in the treatment group, as compared to those who received placebo. Moreover, biochemical measurements revealed a significant increase in 25-OHD concentrations and decrease in serum parathyroid hormone level in a treated group. Furthermore, the beneficial effects on hip and non-vertebral fracture rates was retained after a further eighteen months of treatment (Chapuy *et al.* 1994). The effective prevention of fractures obtained with vitamin D supplementation is not only evident in institutionalised elderly women but also in free-living healthy elderly women and men (Dawson-Hughes *et al.* 1997). In that study, Dawson-Hughes *et al.* were also able to demonstrate a significant reduction in the rate of non-vertebral fractures in a group of men and women, living at home, who received a combination of vitamin D (700 IU/day) and calcium (500 mg/day). Furthermore, despite mean baseline 25-OHD levels of 72 nmol/L in women (compared to the study by Chapuy *et al.* (1992) where mean 25-OHD levels were 24 nmol/L), supplementation resulted in a 33 per cent drop in mean serum PTH level. However, the relative contribution of vitamin D and calcium supplementation in suppressing PTH secretion and decreasing fracture rate is unknown.

In contrast, some studies have failed to show any anti-fracture effects of vitamin D. In a series involving 799 older men and women, 40 per cent of whom were in residential care and the remainder free-living, a single annual injection of 150,000–300,000 IU of vitamin D for two to five years decreased the risk of long bone fractures (upper limbs and ribs); however, there was no apparent protection against hip fracture (Heikinheimo *et al.* 1992). Likewise, Lips *et al.* (1996) studied the effect of 400 IU daily of vitamin D (cholecalciferol) substitution on BMD and fracture rate in a prospective, double blind trial in 2,578 elderly men and women, with a mean age of 80 years. Unlike the Chapuy study, no calcium supplement was used and 40 per cent of the subjects in the Lips' study lived independently. After a median follow-up of 42 months vitamin D supplementation produced no beneficial effect and there was no reduction in fracture rate.

As with the effects of vitamin D metabolites on BMD (as discussed earlier), there is also controversy over the anti-fracture effect. Similar to the data on bone mineral density, controlled trials have been conducted in patients with osteoporosis. Trials with alfacalcidiol (1-alpha-hydroxyvitamin D3) have shown a reduction in vertebral fracture rate (Shiraki *et al.* 1985; Orimo *et al.* 1994); other studies have failed to show a beneficial effect on fracture rate (Christiansen *et al.* 1980; Menczel *et al.* 1995). It must be noted that the beneficial effects of alfacalcidiol reported by Shiraki *et al.* (1985) were not sustained after interruption of the treatment. Similar controversy has been noted in trial using calcitriol. In the largest randomised trial of calcitriol, a controlled study in 622 post-menopausal women with osteoporotic vertebral fractures, 0.25 mcg of calcitriol given twice daily resulted in fewer vertebral fractures compared to the controlled group which received 1g of calcium daily (Tilyard *et al.* 1992). Similar beneficial effects have been reported by Gallagher *et al.* (1989). Others have not been able to demonstrate a beneficial effect of calcitriol on fracture outcome (Christiansen *et al.* 1981; Ott & Chesnut 1989). Treatment with calcitriol, in particular high doses (>0.5 mcg/day), is associated with an increased risk of hypercalcuria and hypercalcaemia (Aloia *et al.* 1988), and close monitoring of serum calcium level is essential.

So how does one explain these controversial findings in the literature, regarding both vitamin D and vitamin D metabolites. In the randomised studies by Chapuy *et al.* (1992) and Dawson-Hughes *et al.* (1997), the dose of vitamin D was 800 IU and 700 IU per day respectively, whilst the dose in the study by Lips *et al.* (1996) was 400 IU per day. It is possible that the higher dose of vitamin D may be responsible for the differences in clinical outcome. As discussed earlier there is an inverse relationship between changes in PTH and changes in bone mineral density. The studies by Chapuy *et al.* and Dawson-Hughes *et al.* demonstrated a significant reduction in PTH levels, whereas the study by Lips *et al.*, which failed to demonstrate any anti-fracture benefit, did not show a significant decrease in serum PTH concentrations. Furthermore, the mean baseline 25-OHD levels in the study by Dawson-Hughes *et al.* was 72 nmol/L, a level which would otherwise be classified as normal by many authors. Despite this level of 25-OHD, the authors were able to show that 700 IU per day of vitamin D produced a 33 per cent drop in serum PTH levels, with an increase in bone mineral density and a reduction in fracture rates. It has therefore been suggested that serum 25-OHD levels need to be maintained at 110 nmol/L (see above) in order to prevent secondary hyperparathyroidism (Dawson-Hughes *et al.* 1997). Another important factor, which may have accounted for the differences seen in these studies, is the daily dietary calcium intake. In the studies by Chapuy *et al.* and Dawson-Hughes *et al.*, the mean daily calcium intake was 513 mg per day and 725 mg per day, respectively, compared to 1,000 mg per day in the study by Lips *et al.* It could be argued that, although vitamin D supplementation is necessary to reverse vitamin D deficiency and insufficiency, an adequate calcium intake is even more important for the skeleton given that the major skeletal defect is calcium deficiency.

Similarly the differences noted in the studies using vitamin D metabolites might be explained in terms of customary dietary intakes, where the positive studies seem to come from countries with low calcium intakes, such as Japan. The differences in the clinical studies involving vitamin D metabolites, as mentioned above, may not only be accounted for by the differences in dietary calcium or vitamin D status, but also by the differences in the vitamin D receptor (VDR) genotype, in particular in elderly subjects. The exact mechanism by which VDR genotype may influence calcium homeostasis remains to be clarified. However, current evidence suggests that the BB genotype in women is strongly associated with low bone mass (Morrison *et al.* 1994), accelerated bone loss (Krall *et al.* 1995), and woman with the BB genotype have blunted calcium absorption during calcium restriction (Dawson-Hughes *et al.* 1993).

Conclusion

Calcium intake is positively correlated with bone mass at all ages. A need for a higher calcium intake and calcium supplementation is particularly important during adolescence where it plays one of the major roles in achieving peak bone mass and for women after the menopause, where increased calcium intake/supplementation reduces the rate of age- related bone loss. Although the studies are limited, it is apparent that long-term calcium supplementation has benefits in terms of reduction of fracture risk.

In the elderly, vitamin D deficiency/insufficiency is an endemic problem and plays a part in the pathogenesis of osteopaenia/osteoporosis. There is a strong case for routine vitamin D supplementation in high-risk subjects. For example, in those with a low calcium dietary intake, absence of exposure to sunlight, in those with low femoral bone densities and in particular in individuals where there is a low serum 25-OHD and high serum PTH concentration, such as the elderly and Asian immigrants. Finally, provided that dietary calcium intakes are adequate (Table 6.1), then a case can be made for vitamin D supplementation alone, given that the effects of both vitamin D and calcium are thought to occur primarily through a reduction in PTH mediated bone loss.

References

Aaron JE, Gallagher JC, Nordin BEC (1974). Seasonal variation of histological osteomalacia in femoral neck fractures. *Lancet* **ii,** 84–6.

Aloia JF, Vaswani A, Yeh J, Ellis K, Yasumara S, Cohn S (1988). Calcitriol in the treatment of postmenopausal osteoporosis. *Am J Med* **84,** 401–8.

Aloia JF, Vaswani A, Yeh JK, Ross PL, Flaster E, Dilmanian FA (1994). Calcium supplementation with and without hormone replacement therapy to prevent postmenopausal bone loss. *Ann Int Med* **120,** 97–103.

Baran D, Sorenson A, Grimes J *et al.* (1990). Dietary modification with diary products for preventing vertebral bone loss in premenopausal women: a three year prospective study. *J Clin Endorinol Metab* **70,** 264–70.

Bauer DC, Browner WS, Cauley JA *et al.* (1993). Factors associated with appendicular bone mass in older women. *Ann Int Med* **118,** 657–65.

Bell NH (1985). Vitamin D-endocrine system. *J Clin Invest* **76,** 1–6.

Blumsohn A, Herrington K, Hannon RA *et al.* (1994). The effect of calcium on the circadian rhythm of bone resorption. *J Clin Endocrinol Metab* **79,** 730–35.

Bonjour J-P, Theintz G, Buchs B, Slosman D, Rizzoli R (1991). Critical years and stages of puberty for spinal and femoral bone mass accumulation during adolescence. *J Clin Endocrinology Metab* **73,** 555–63.

Breslau NA (1996). Calcium, magnesium, and phosphorus: Intestinal absorption. In: *Primer on the Metabolic Bone Diseases and Disorders of Mineral Metabolism. Third Edition.* London: Lippincott-Raven, pp. 41–49.

Burns J & Paterson CR (1985). Single dose vitamin D treatment for osteomalacia in the elderly. *BMJ* **290,** 281–282.

Cadogan J, Eastell R, Jones N, Barker ME (1997). Milk intake and bone mineral acquisition in adolescent girls: randomised, controlled intervention trial. *BMJ* **315,** 1255–60.

Chan GM, Hess M, Hollis J, Book LS (1984). Bone mineral status in childhood accidental fractures. *Am J Dis Child* **38,** 569–70.

Chapuy MC, Arlot ME, Delmas PD, Meunier PJ (1994). Effect of calcium and cholecalciferol treatment for three years on hip fractures in elderly women. *BMJ* **308,** 1081–82.

Chapuy MC, Arlot M, Duboeuf F *et al.* (1992). Vitamin D3 and calcium to prevent hip fractures in elderly women. *N Engl J Med* **327,** 1637–42.

Chapuy M, Chapuy P, Meunier P (1987). Calcium and vitamin D supplements: effects on calcium metabolism in elderly people. *Am J Clin Nutr* **46,** 324–28.

Chevalley T, Rizzoli R, Nydegger V *et al.* (1994). Effects of calcium supplementation on femoral bone mineral density and vertebral fracture rate in vitamin-D-replete elderly patients. *Osteoporosis Int* **4,** 245–52.

Christiansen C, Christensen MS, McNair P, Hagen C, Stocklumd K, Transbol JB (1980). Prevention of early postmenopausal bone loss: controlled 2-year study in 315 normal females. *Eur J Clin Invest* **10,** 273–9.

Christiansen C, Christensen MS, Rodbro P, Hagen C, Transbol JB (1981). Effect of 1,25-dihydroxyvitamin D3 in itself or combined with hormone treatment in preventing postmenopausal osteoporosis. *Eur J Clin Invest* **11,** 305–9.

Compston JE (1995). The role of vitamin D and calcium supplementation in the prevention of osteoporotic fractures in the elderly. *Clin Enocrinol* **43,** 393–405.

Cumming RG (1990). Calcium intake and bone mass: a quantitative review of the evidence. *Calcif Tiss Int* **47,** 194–201.

Cummings SR, Black DM, Nevitt MC *et al.* (1990). Appendicular bone density and age predict hip fracture in women. *JAMA* **263**, 665-8.

Cummings SR, Nevitt M, Browner W *et al.* (1995). Risk factors for hip fracture in white women. *N Engl J Med* **332**, 767–73.

Dawson-Hughes B (1993). Calcium supplementation and bone loss: a review of controlled clinical trials. *Am J Clin Nutr* **54**, S274–80.

Dawson-Hughes B, Dallal GE, Krall EA, Harris S, Sokoll LJ, Falconer G (1991). Effect of vitamin D supplemntation on wintertime and overall bone loss in healthy postmenopausal women. *Ann Int Med* **115**, 505–12.

Dawson-Hughes B, Dallal G, Krall E *et al.* (1990). A controlled trial of the effect of calcium supplementation on bone density in postmenopausal women. *N Engl J Med* **323**, 878–83.

Dawson-Hughes B, Harris SS, Dallal GT (1997). Plasma calcidiol, season and parathyroid hormone concentrations in healthy elderly men and women. *Am J Clin Nutr* **65**, 67–71.

Dawson-Hughes B, Harris SS, Finneran S (1995). Calcium absorption on high and low calcium intakes in relation to vitamin D receptor genotype. *J Clin Endocrin Metab* **80**, 3657–3661.

Dawson-Hughes B, Harris SS, Krall EA, Dallal GE (1997). Effect of calcium and vitamin D supplementation on bone density in men and women 65 years of age or older. *N Engl J Med* **337**, 701–2.

Dawson-Hughes B, Harris SS, Krall EA, Dallal GE, Falconer G, Green CL (1995). Rates of bone loss in postmenopausal women randomly assigned to one of two dosages of vitamin D. *Am J Clin Nutr* **61**, 1140–5.

Department of Health (1989). *The Diets of British Schoolchildren.* (*Report on Health and Social Subjects No 36*). London: HMSO.

Elders PJ, Lips P, Netelenbos JC *et al.* (1994). Long-term effect of calcium supplementation on bone loss in perimenopausal women. *J Bone Miner Res* **9**, 963–70.

Fujita T (1990). Studies of osteoporosis in Japan. *Metabolism* **39**, S39–42.

Gallagher ME, Riggs BL, Recker RR, Goldgar D (1989). The effects of calcitriol on patients with postmenopausal osteoporosis with special reference to fracture frequency. *Proc Soc Exp Biol Med* **191**, 287–92.

Heaney RP (1986). Calcium, bone health and osteoporosis. *Bone Miner Res* **4**, 255–301.

Heaney RP (1991). Calcium supplements: practical considerations. *Osteoporosis Int* **1**, 65-71.

Heaney RP (1995) Skeletal development and maintenance: The role of calcium and vitamin D. In: *Advances in Endocrinology and metabolism* **6**, 17–38.

Heaney RP (1996). Nutrition and risk for osteoporosis. In: *Osteoporosis* San Diego: Academic Press, pp 483–505.

Heaney RP, Recker RR, Stegman MR, Moy AJ (1989). Calcium absorption in women: relationships to calcium intake, estrogen status, and age. *J Bone Min Res* **4**, 469–75.

Heikinheimo RJ, Inkovaara JA, Harju EJ *et al.* (1992). Annual injection of vitamin D and fractures of aged bones. *Calcif Tissue Int* **51**, 105–10.

Heshmati HM, Khosla S, Burritt MF, O'Fallan WM, Riggs BL (1998). A defect in renal calcium conservation may contribute to the pathogenesis of postmenopausal osteoporosis. *J Clin Endocrinology Metab* **83**, 1916–20.

Holbrook TL, Barrett-Connor E, Wingard DL (1998). Dietary calcium and risk of hip fracture: 14-year prospective population study. *Lancet* **ii**, 1046–49.

Holick MF (1995). Noncalcaemic actions of 1,25-dihydroxyvitamin D3 and clinical applications. *Bone* **17**, S107–111.

Holick MF (1994). Vitamin D: New horizons for the 21st century. *Am J Clin Nutr* **60,** 619–30.

Holick MF (1995). Vitamin D: Photobiology, metabolism, and clinical applications. In DeGroot L *et al.* (eds): *Endocrinology. Third Edition,* Philadelphia: WB Saunders, pp 990–1013

Holick MF, Matsuoka LY, Wortsman J (1989). Age, Philadelphia: Vitamin D, and solar ultraviolet radiation. *Lancet* **iv,** 1104–5.

Jackman LA, Millane SS, Martin BR *et al.* (1997). Calcium retention in relation to calcium intake and postmenarcheal age in adolescent females. *Am J Clin Nutr* **66,** 327–33.

Johnston CC, Miller JZ, Slemenda CE *et al.* (1992). Calcium supplementation and increases in bone mineral density in children. *N Engl J Med* **327,** 82–7.

Kanis J, Johnell O, Gulborg B *et al.* (1992). Evidence for efficacy of drugs affecting bone metabolism in preventing hip fractures. *BMJ* **305,** 1124–28.

Khaw KT, Sneyd MT, Compston J (1992). Bone density, parathyroid hormone and 25 hydroxyvitamin D concentration in middle-aged women. *BMJ* **305,** 273–9.

Kooh SW, Frazer D, Reilly BJ, Hamilton JR, Gall DG, Bell L (1977). Rickets due to calcium deficiency. *N Engl J Med* **297,** 1264–6.

Krall EA, Parry P, Lichter JB, Dawson-Hughes B (1995). Vitamin D receptor alleles and rates of bone loss: influences of years since menopause and calcium intake. *J Bone Min Res* **10,** 978–984.

Krall E, Sahyoun N, Tannenbaum S, Dallal G, Dawson-Hughes B (1989). Effect of vitamin D intake on seasonal variations in parathyroid hormone secretion in post-menopausal women. *N Engl J Med* **321,** 1777–83.

Lau EMC, Woo J, Leung PC, Swaminathan R, Leung D (1992). The effects of calcium supplementation and exercise on bone density in elderly Chinese women. *Osteoporosis Int* **2,** 168–73.

Lee WT, Leung SS, Leung DM, Chen JC (1996). A follow-up study on the effects of calcium-supplement withdrawal and puberty on bone acquisition of children. *Am J Clin Nutr* **64,** 71–77.

Lee WTK, Leung SS, Lui SSH, Lau J (1993). Relationship between long term calcium intake and bone mineral content of children aged from birth to 5 years. *Br J Nutr* **70,** 235–48.

Lee WTK, Leung SSF, Ng M-Y *et al.* (1993). Bone mineral content of two populations of Chinese children with different calcium intakes. *Bone Miner* **23,** 195–206.

Lee WTK, Leung SS, Wang SH *et al.* (1994) Double-blind controlled calcium supplementation and bone mineral accretion in children accustomed to a low-calcium diet. *Am J Clin Nutr* **60,** 744–50.

Lips P, Graafmans WC, Ooms ME, Bezemer PD, Bouter LM (1996). Vitamin D supplementation and fracture incidence in elderly persons: a randomised placebo-controlled clinical trial. *Ann Intern Med* **124,** 400–6.

Lips P, Wiersinga A, van Ginkel FC, Jongen MJM *et al.* (1988). The effect of vitamin D supplementation on vitamin D status and parathyroid function in elderly subjects. *J Clin Endocrinol Metab* **67,** 644–70.

Lloyd T, Andon MB, Rollings N *et al.* (1993). Calcium supplementation and bone mineral density in adolescent girls. *JAMA* **270,** 841–4.

Long RG, Skinner RK, Meinhard E *et al.* (1976). Serum 25-hydroxyvitamin D values in liver disease and hepatic osteomalacia. *Gut* **17,** 824–27.

Looker AC, Harris TB, Madans JH, Sempos CT (1993). Dietary calcium and hip fracture risk: the NHANES I epidemiology follow-up study. *Osteoporosis Int* **3,** 177–84.

Lukert B, Higgins J, Stoskopf M (1992). Menopausal bone loss is partially regulated by dietary intake of vitamin D. *Calcif Tissue Int* **51**, 173–9.

Matkovic V & Heaney RP (1992) Calcium balance during human growth: evidence for threshold behaviour. *Am J Clin Nutr* **55**, 992–6.

Matkovic V, Fontana D, Tominac C, Goel P, Chestnut CH III (1990). Factors that influence peak bone mass formation: a study of calcium balance and the inheritance of bone mass in adolescent females. *Am J Clin Nutr* **52**, 878–8.

Matkovic V, Jelic T, Wardlaw GM *et al.* (1994). Timing of peak bone mass in caucasian females and its implications for the prevention of osteoporosis. *J Clin Invest* **93**, 799–808.

Matkovic V, Kostial K, Simonovic I, Brodarec A, Buzina R (1977). Influence of calcium intake, age and sex on bone. *Calcific Tissue Res* **22**, 393–96.

Matkovic V, Kostial K, Simonovic I, Buzina R, Brodarec A, Nordin BEC (1979). Bone status and fracture rates in two regions of Yugoslavia. *Am J Clin Nutr* **32**, 540–9.

McKane WR, Khosla S, O'Fallon WM, Robins SP, Burritt MF, Riggs BL (1996). Role of calcium intake in modulating age-related increases in parathyroid function and bone resorption. *J Clin Endocrinol Metab* **81**, 1699–1703.

McKenna MJ (1992). Differences in vitamin D status between countries in young adults and the elderly. *Am J Med* **93**, 69–77.

McKenna MJ & Freaney R (1997). Defining hypovitaminosis D in the elderly. In Burckhardt P, Dawson-Hughes B, Heaney RP (eds); *Nutritional Aspects of Osteoporosis* New York: Springer.

McKenna MJ, Freaney R (1998). Secondary hyperparathyroidism in the elderly: Means to defining hypovitaminosis D. *Osteoporosis Int* **8**, S3–6.

Menczel J, Foldes J, Steinberg R *et al.* (1995). Alfacalcidol (alpha D3) and calcium osteoporosis. *Clin Orthop* **300**, 241–7.

Morrison NA, Qi JC, Tokita A *et al.* (1994). Prediction of bone density from vitamin D receptor alleles. *Nature* **367**, 284–87.

Murphy S, Khaw K-T, May H, Compston JE (1994). Milk consumption and bone mineral density in middle aged elderly women. *BMJ* **308**, 939–41.

Nicar MJ & Pak CYC (1985). Calcium bioavailability from calcium carbonate and calcium citrate. *J Clin Endocrinol Metab* **61**, 391–93.

NIH Consensus Conference (1994). Optimal Calcium Intake. *JAMA* **272**, 1942–48.

Nordin BEC (1997). Calcium and osteoporosis. *Nutrition* **13**, 664–86.

Ooms ME, Roos JC, Bezemer PD, Van der Vijgh WJF, Bouter LM, Lips P (1995). prevention of bone loss by vitamin D supplementation in elderly women: a randomised double-blind trial. *J Clin Endocrinol Metab* **80**, 1052–8.

Orimo H, Shiraki M, Hatashi Y *et al.* (1994). Effects of 1 alpha-hydroxyvitamin D3 on lumbar bone mineral density and vertebral fractures in patients with postmenopausal osteoporosis. *Calcif Tissue Int* **54**, 370–76.

Orr JB (1928). Milk consumption and the growth of school children. *Lancet* **i**, 202–13.

Ott SM (1991) Bone density in adolescents. *N Engl J Med* **325**, 1646–7.

Ott SM & Chestnut CH (1989). Calcitriol treatment is not effective in postmenopausal osteoporosis. *Ann Int Med* **110**, 267–74.

Paganini-Hill A, Chao A, Ross RK, Henderson BE (1991). Exercise and other factors in the prevention of hip fracture: the Leisure World Study. *Epidemiology* **2**, 16–25.

Pak CYC, Breslau NA, Harvey JA (1986). Nutrition and metabolic bone disease. *In Nutritional Diseases: Research Directions in Comparative Pathobiology* Alan R Liss pp 215–40.

Parfitt AM, Gallagher JC, Heaney RP, Johnson CC, Neer P, Whedon G (1982). Vitamin D and bone disease in the elderly. *Am J Clin Nutr* **36**, 1014–31.

Pietrek J & Kokot F (1977). Serum 25-hydroxyvitamin D in patients with chronic renal disease. *Eur J Clin Invest* **7**, 283–87.

Prestwood K, Pannullo A, Kenny A *et al.* (1996). The effect of a short course of calcium and vitamin D on bone turnover in older women. *Osteoporosis Int* **6**, 314–19.

Recker RR (1985). Calcium absorption and achlorhydria. *N Eng J Med* **73**, 70–3.

Recker RR, Davies KM, Hinders SM *et al.* (1992). Bone gain in young adult women. *JAMA* **268**, 2403–08.

Recker RR, Hinders S, Davies KM *et al.* (1996). Correcting calcium nutritional deficiency prevents spine fractures in elderly women. *J Bone Miner Res* **11**, 1961–6.

Reid DM & New SA (1997). Nutritional influences on bone mass. *Proc Nutr Soc* **50**, 977–87.

Reid IR, Ames RW, Evans MI *et al.* (1993). Effect of calcium supplementation on bone loss in postmenopausal women. *N Engl J Med* **328**, 460–64.

Reid IR, Ames RW, Evans MC *et al.* (1995). Long-term effects of calcium supplementation on bone loss and fractures in postmenopausal women: a randomised controlled trial. *Am J Clin Nutr* **98**, 331–35.

Rico H, Revilla M, Villa LF *et al.* (1994). Longitudinal study of the effect of calcium pidolate on bone mass in eugonadal women. *Calcif Tiss Int* **54**, 477–80.

Sambrook P, Birmingham J, Kelly P *et al.* (1993). Prevention of corticosteroid osteoporosis. A comparison of calcium, calcitriol and calcitonin. *N Engl J Med* **328**, 1747–52.

Sandler RB, Slemenda CW, LaPorte RE *et al.* (1995). Postmenopausal bone density and milk consumption in childhood and adolescence. *Am J Clin Nutr* **42**, 270–4.

Shiraki M, Orimo H, Ito H *et al.* (1985). Long-term treatment of postmenopausal osteoporosis with active vitamin D_3, 1-alpha-hydroxycholecalciferol (1alpha-OHD$_3$) and 1,24-dihydroxycholecalciferol (1,24(OH)$_2$D$_3$). *Endocrin Jap* **32**, 305–15.

Slemenda C, Reister TK, Peacock M, Johnston CC (1993). Bone growth in children following cessation of calcium supplementation. *J Bone Min Res* **8**, S154.

Smith E, Gilligan C, Smith P, Surpos C (1989). Calcium supplementation and bone loss in middle aged women. *Am J Clin Nutr* **50**, 833–42.

Teegarden D, Proulx WR, Martin BR *et al.* (1995) Peak bone mass in young women. *J Bone Miner Res* **10**, 711–5.

Thomas MK, Llyod-Jones DM, Thadhani RI *et al.* (1998). Hypovitaminosis in medical inpatients. *N Engl J Med* **338**, 777–83.

Tilyard MW, Spears GFS, Thomson J, Dovey S (1992). Treatment of postmenopausal osteoporosis with calcitriol or calcium. *N Engl J Med* **326**, 357–62.

Warady BD, Lindsley CB, Robinson FG, Lukert BP (1994). Effects of nutritional supplementation on bone mineral status of children with rheumatic diseases receiving corticosteroid therapy. *J Rheum* **21**, 530–35.

Wickham CA, Walsh K Cooper *et al.* (1989). Dietary calcium, physical activity, and risk of hip fracture: a prospective study. *BMJ* **299**, 889–92.

Chapter 7

The role of hormone replacement therapy and the skeletal role of the selective oestrogen receptor modulators: issues of use and concordance

Janice Rymer

Hormone replacement therapy (HRT) is prescribed to relieve the acute symptoms of oestrogen deficiency and to prevent the longterm consequences of ovarian failure. HRT prevents bone loss from the female skeleton after the menopause and maintains the bone mass for the duration of treatment in the majority of women (Christiansen *et al.* 1980). After ovarian failure there is increased bone remodelling and the rate of bone loss is accelerated. Although the precise mechanism is not clear, oestrogen probably acts through some form of steroid receptor mechanism (Bland 2000).

Despite the convincing evidence that HRT protects the post-menopausal skeleton from bone loss, (Lindsay *et al.* 1976; Horsman *et al.* 1977; Recker *et al.* 1977; Christiansen *et al.* 1980) adherence to date has been poor. The issue of adherence is complex, involving patient factors, doctor factors, the medication itself and other factors. The patient factors involve the decision to seek healthcare, the expectation of the consultation and the expectation of the prescription. The initial decision to seek healthcare is influenced by women's previous experiences and pre-existing attitudes. Whether or not she takes the medication revolves around her understanding of the need for therapy, but this is influenced by experiences of her friends and relatives and what she has read in the media. As physicians, we would assume that women would be concerned in the longterm with the medical consequences of ovarian failure. However, Graziottin (1996) found that women were concerned much more with self-image and sexual identity and this was more motivating with regard to taking HRT than unknown medical consequences. Clearly, when talking about ovarian failure, the experience of symptoms will change a woman's attitude as to whether or not she will take HRT. Quite simply, if she is not feeling well and feels better on HRT, then she will be more inclined to take therapy. Therefore surveying pre-menopausal women about whether or not they will take HRT post-menopausally is not a true reflection of what will happen if they are not motivated by experiencing negative symptoms. With regard to the doctor factors, this involves the doctor's knowledge of the condition and his confidence and competence in managing the post-menopausal woman.

The pharmaceutical industry has now supplied us with a vast range of preparations and adherence will depend on the convenience of the drug, and the perceived side-effects.

Other factors include the influence of the media, the availability of information leaflets and the experiences of friends and relatives.

HRT preparations available

The diversity of current HRT preparations is now overwhelming and illustrates the fact that no one preparation will suit all women. However, despite the range of preparations the number of women taking HRT and remaining on it is still low. There remains reluctance on the part of GPs to prescribe HRT and on the part of women to take it (Spector 1989). Only 9 per cent of post-menopausal women in London (Garnett *et al.* 1991) and 3 per cent in Glasgow (Barlow *et al.* 1989) received HRT for more than three years. Ryan and colleagues (1992) reported a group of post-menopausal women who self-referred for bone density screening and were found to have low bone density. They were therefore at risk of developing osteoporosis and were advised to take HRT. However, at eight months only 60 per cent of these women were still receiving HRT. One of the major reasons in this study for discontinuation of treatment was the return to monthly bleeding. At the time when the study was performed there were no non-bleeding therapies available. However, we now have four regimes for non-bleeding therapy, listed below:

- Continuous combined therapies where oestrogen and progestogens are given continuously and the continuous low dose progestogen opposes the action of oestrogen on the endometrium so that the endometrium is not stimulated
- Oestrogen replacement therapy and the progestogen intra-uterine system. With this regime the progestogen is released locally daily from the intra-uterine device so that it acts primarily at the endometrial surface inducing an atrophic endometrium. The oestrogen can then be given by any route
- Tibolone is a synthetic compound that exhibits oestrogenic, progestogenic, and androgenic properties. The delta 4 isomer, one of the major metabolites, predominates at the level of the endometrium and exerts a progestogenic influence inducing an atrophic endometrium
- Selective Oestrogen Receptor Modulators (SERMs) – not strictly speaking a form of HRT, but they are a non-bleeding therapy to protect the female skeleton. They will be discussed later in this chapter.

Undoubtedly, with the introduction of non-bleeding therapies, adherence will be improved. Three two-year studies investigating the effects of tibolone on the female skeleton had a 70 per cent adherence rate after two years (Rymer *et al.* 1994; Studd *et al.* 1996; Bjarnason *et al.* 1997). This is significantly higher compared to other bone studies using conventional HRT.

How to increase adherence?

The issues of side-effects, women's fears regarding taking HRT and education are discussed below.

Side-effects

The commonest side-effects experienced by women are vaginal bleeding problems, breast tenderness, nausea, oedema, and weight gain. Break through bleeding is common with continuous combined therapy (25 per cent–50 per cent in the first six months) and with tibolone (10 per cent–20 per cent in the first six months) (Rymer *et al.* 1994). The management of these bleeding episodes is quite straight forward and much easier with the introduction of transvaginal ultrasound scanning, outpatient endometrial sampling and hysteroscopy. If bleeding occurs in the first six months of therapy no further management is needed unless there is a high index of suspicion in an individual woman that there may have been underlying endometrial pathology prior to commencement of therapy, for example, obesity, diabetes, or polycystic ovarian syndrome. If bleeding occurs after six months then investigation is warranted (Spencer & Whitehead 1999). With transvaginal scanning a good view of the endometrial echo can be obtained and endometrial thickness can be measured. If the thickness is greater than 5 mm an endometrial assessment is needed, either with an endometrial biopsy or with outpatient hysteroscopy. If an adequate biopsy can be obtained with an outpatient sampler and histology is normal, the woman can continue with the non-bleeding therapy and a transvaginal scan repeated in six months if she has further bleeding. If an endometrial biopsy cannot be obtained an outpatient hysteroscopy should be performed with some form of local anaesthetic to the cervix to allow dilatation. Further management will depend on the results of these investigations (Spencer & Whitehead 1999).

When commencing a woman on a non-bleeding therapy such as continuous combined or tibolone it is worth restricting the use to post-menopausal women who are one year past their last menstrual period. It is not harmful to introduce these therapies earlier but there may be significantly more episodes of breakthrough bleeding and this will negatively influence compliance rates (Urlich *et al.* 1997). If there is uncertainty about the last menstrual period (for example if the woman has been on sequential HRT for months or years) then one needs to concentrate carefully on the history and enquire into the woman's age, why HRT was commenced initially, and for how long she has been on the therapy. If in doubt one could try a continuous combined therapy or tibolone for six months; further management will depend on the incidence of break through bleeding (Rymer 1998).

If a woman has not been exposed to oestrogen for 12 months she may experience significant breast tenderness and engorgement on commencing any form of oestrogen (Domoney & Studd 2000). This should settle down after the first three months when all the hormonal receptors will be saturated but it may be worth starting her on a very low dose of HRT and gradually increasing over three months until she is at a bone sparing dose. Nausea is usually a transient problem and should settle down over a few weeks. Some women develop idiopathic oedema on HRT but this is a very small percentage.

Women perceive that they gain weight on HRT but studies do not support this. Women of this age group tend to gain weight and this will not be altered by the HRT (Kritz-Silverstein & Barrett-Connor 1996). This is a very important message to get across to women and they need to concentrate more on lifestyle changes such as diet and exercise to counteract what appears to be a natural phenomenon.

Women's fears

Women's major concern with HRT is its effect on the breast. Many women perceive that breast cancer is the major killer of women. Breast tissue is oestrogen sensitive and oestrogen stimulates breast tumour cells in vitro. The latest meta-analysis has shown that longterm treatment (greater than five years) does lead to an increase in the relative risk of breast cancer by a factor of 1.023 for each year of use. (Collaborative Group 1997). Put another way, if 1,000 women use HRT for ten years starting at age 50, it is estimated that, by the age of 70, there will be an additional six cases of breast cancer raising the background incidence from 45 to 51 cases. The limited data suggest use of progestogens has not diminished the excess risk associated with oestrogens.

Women are also concerned that HRT may induce endometrial carcinoma. Unopposed oestrogen will increase the incidence of endometrial hyperplasia and carcinoma. Progestogens substantially decrease the excess risk of endometrial cancer but must either be taken for 12–14 days of each month or continuously (Studd et al. 1980; Whitehead et al. 1982).

Women on HRT appear to have an increased relative risk of three times of venous thromboembolic disease compared to women who are not on HRT (Daly et al. 1996; Jick et al. 1996). However the absolute risk is low in the order of three in ten thousand. The increase in risk appears to be restricted to the first year of use with an odds ratio of 4.6 (95 per cent CI 2.5–8.4) during the first six months. This suggests that HRT may be unmasking an underlying thrombophilia (Bertina & Rosendaal 1998).

Education

Women need to be informed of the side-effects they may encounter prior to commencing HRT and their concerns must be discussed. As physicians we need to be clear about the contraindications.

The HRT data sheets inaccurately list the contraindications, most of which have been extrapolated from oral contraceptive data. This is unfortunate as the alkyl oestrogens are very different from the esterised or micronised oestrogens used in HRT. Absolute contraindications are pregnancy, active venous thromboembolism, severe active liver disease and endometrial and breast cancer with recurrence. Relative contraindications are abnormal vaginal bleeding, breast lump, previous endometrial and breast carcinoma, strong family history of breast cancer and previous venous thromboembolism. However with both the absolute and relative contraindications one must always weigh up the risk versus quality of life (Rymer 2000).

Selective oestrogen receptor modulators

Selective oestrogen receptor modulators (SERMs) are a group of antioestrogens that possess agonistic activity on some tissues and antagonist activity on other tissues. Clomiphene was the first antioestrogen to be developed and was originally found to act as a post-coital contraceptive agent in rats (Spencer *et al.* 1999). In later years this compound was used as an adjunct in the treatment of anovulatory infertility. Tamoxifen, a related antioestrogen, has been used as adjuvant treatment for pre- and post-menopausal women with oestrogen receptor positive breast cancer (Harper & Walpole 1967; Lobsetwar 1970). Raloxifene, a non-steroidal compound derived from a benzothiophene series of antioestrogens, has now been released for use in post-menopausal women to prevent bone loss in the spine and femoral neck, and, more recently, has been shown to reduce vertebral fracture (Ettinger *et al.* 1999). The biochemical markers of bone metabolism suggest that the mode of action on the bone remodelling unit is very similar to that of oestrogen (Delmas *et al.* 1997). To date there are no clinical fracture data. With regard to the cardiovascular system, raloxifene has a mixed effect with a probable overall beneficial effect but again clinical end point data are awaiting. Raloxifene does not eliminate the vasomotor symptoms or urogenital symptoms of oestrogen deficiency (Fuchs-Young *et al.* 1995). Raloxifene does not stimulate endometrial proliferation and the reports of vaginal bleeding are no more frequent than controls. The appealing feature of raloxifene is that it does appear to decrease the relative risk of developing breast cancer. The American Society of Clinical Oncology has demonstrated the rate of breast cancer in controls was that expected from the population studies and that the observed deficit in breast cancer in the raloxifene-treated group was among oestrogen receptor positive tumours. It was suggested that raloxifene acts as an antagonist on breast tissue (Cummings *et al.* 1999).

Raloxifene will not relieve the vasomotor symptoms produced by oestrogen deficiency and some women may experience vasomotor symptoms as a side-effect of the compound. Raloxifene does not have beneficial effects on the urogential tract so women symptomatic of vaginal dryness or dyspareunia will not benefit from the SERMs. Therefore the place of the SERMs is probably for post-menopausal women who are not suffering from vasomotor symptoms or vaginal dryness, who want to protect their skeleton and who are concerned about the risk of developing breast cancer. This would suggest that the SERMs would be ideal for the older post-menopausal woman (Purdie & Beardsworth 1991).

Summary

If women are suffering from the acute symptoms of oestrogen deficiency, then HRT will improve their quality of life. If they are concerned about developing osteoporosis, then HRT or the SERMs will have a beneficial effect on the bone. Women's main concern is the development of breast cancer and it does appear that the incidence of breast cancer is increased when women take HRT. However this must be put into perspective and women are much more likely to die of cardiovascular disease than breast cancer. If comparing HRT to the SERMs, then HRT will be beneficial as far as oestrogen-deficient symptoms go. The SERMs will be beneficial if women are concerned about developing breast cancer. Adherence remains a significant problem, and if women do not like HRT, or they are concerned about the side-effects or the longterm risks then they will not take it.

Therefore to increase adherence we need to address the issues of side-effects, concerns with HRT and education of women, the media, and the medical profession.

References

Barlow DH, Grosset KA, Hart H, Hart DM (1989). A study of the experience of Glasgow women in the climacteric years. *Br J Obstet Gynecol* **96**, 1192–97.

Bertina RM & Rosendaal FR (1998). Venous thrombosis. The interaction of genes and environment. *New England Journal of Medicine* **338**, 1840–1.

Bjarnason NH, Bjarnason K, Haarbo J *et al.* (1997). Tibolone: prevention of bone loss in late menopausal women. *J Clin Endocrinol Metab* **81**, 2419–22.

Bland R (2000). Steroid hormone receptor expression and action in bone. *Clinical Science* **98**, 217–40.

Christiansen C, Christiansen MF, McNair P, Hagan C, Stockland K-E, Tranbol IB (1980). Prevention of postmenopausal bone: controlled two year study in 315 normal females. *Eur J Clin Inves* **10**, 273–279.

Collaborative Group on Hormonal Factors in Breast Cancer (1997). Breast cancer and hormone replacement therapy: collaborative reanalyses of data from 51 epidemiological studies of 52,705 women with breast cancer and 108,411 women without breast cancer. *Lancet* **35**, 1047–59.

Cummings SR, Eckert S, Krueger KA *et al.* (1999). The effect of raloxifene on risk of breast cancer in postmenopausal women: results from the MORE randomised trial. *JAMA* **281**, 2189–2197.

Daly E, Vessey MP, Hawkins MM, Carson JL, Gough P, Marsh S (1996). Risk of venous thromboembolism and users of HRT. *Lancet* **348**, 977–83.

Delmas P, Bjarnason N, Mitlak B *et al.* (1997). Effects of raloxifene on bone mineral density, serum cholesterol concentrations, and uterine endometrium in postmenopausal women. *N Engl J Med* **337**, 1641–7.

Domoney CL & Studd J (2000). *Continuation with Hormone Replacement Therapy in the Management of the Menopause – the Millennium Review.* Parthenon Publishing Group Ltd., London.

Ettinger B, Black DM, Mitlak BH *et al.* (1999). Reduction of vertebral fracture risk in postmenopausal women with osteoporosis treated with raloxifene: results from a three year randomised clinical trial (MORE Investigators). *JAMA* **282**, 637–645.

Fuchs-Young R, Glasebrook AI, Short LL, Draper MW, Rippy MK, Cole HW *et al.* (1995). Raloxifene is a tissue-selective agonist/antagonist that functions through the estrogen receptor. *Ann N Y Acad Sci* **761**, 355–60.

Garnett T, Mitchell A, Studd J (1991). Patterns of referral to a menopausal clinic. *J R Soc Med* **84**, 128–30.

Graziottin A (1996). HRT: the woman's perspective. *International Journal of Gynaecology & Obstetrics* **52**, S11–6

Harper M & Walpole A (1967). Mode of action ICI 46,474 in preventing implantation in rats. *J Reprod Fertil* **13**, 101–19.

Horman A, Gallagher JC, Simpson M, Nordin BEC (1977). Prospective trial of oestrogen and calcium in postmenopausal women. *British Medical Journal* **II**, 789–92.

Jick H, Derby LE, Myers MW, Vasilakis C, Newton KM (1996). Risk of hospital admission for idiopathic venous thromboembolism among users of postmenopausal oestrogen. *Lancet* **348**, 981–3.

Kritz-Silverstein D & Barrett-Connor E (1996). Long-term postmenopausal hormone use, obesity and fat distribution in older women. *JAMA* **275**, 46–49.

Lindsay R, Hart DM, Atkim JM, McDonald EB, Anderson JB, Clark AC (1976). Long-term prevention of postmenopausal osteoporosis by oestrogen: evidence of an increased bone mass after delayed onset of oestrogen treatment. *Lancet* **i**, 1038–41.

Lobsetwar A (1970). Role of estrogen in ovulation: a study using the estrogen antagonist ICI 46,474. *Endocrinology* **87**, 542–51.

Purdie DW & Beardsworth SA (1991). The selective oestrogen receptor modulation: evolution and clinical applications. *British Journal of Clinical Pharmacology* **48**, 785–92.

Recker RR, Salville PD, Heaney RP (1977). Effective oestrogens and calcium carbonate on bone loss in postmenopausal women. *Ann Intern Med* **87**, 649–55.

Ryan P, Harrison R, Blake GM *et al.* (1992). Compliance with HRT after screening for postmenopausal osteoporosis. *Br J Obstet Gynaecol* **99**, 335–8.

Rymer J, Chapman MG, Fogelman I (1994a). Effect of tibolone on postmenopausal bone loss. *Osteoporosis Int* **4**, 314–17.

Rymer J, Fogelman I, Chapman MG (1994b). The incidence of vaginal bleeding with tibolone treatment. *Br J Obstet Gynaecol* **101**, 53–6.

Rymer JM (1998). The effects of tibolone. *Gynaecol Endocrinol* **12**, 213–20.

Rymer J (2000). Relative and absolute contraindications to hormone replacement therapy in the management of the menopause. In The *Millennium Review 2000.* ed. Studd J. Parthenon Publishing Group, London.

Spector TD (1989). Use of oestrogen replacement therapy in high risk groups in the UK. *British Medical Journal* **299**, 1434–1435.

Spencer CP, Morris EP, Rymer JM (1999). Selective estrogen receptor modulators (SERMs)? Women's panacea for the next millenium. *American Journal of Obstetrics & Gynaecology* **180**, 763–70.

Spencer C & Whitehead M (1999). Endometrial assessment revisited. *British Journal of Obstetrics and Gynaecology* **106**, 623–32.

Studd J, Arnala I, Zamblera D *et al.* (1996). Tibolone increases bone mass in women with previous fractures in a placebo controlled bicentre study. *Osteoporosis Int* **6**, 230.

Studd JWW, Thom MH, Patterson MEL, Wade-Evans T (1980). *The Prevention and Treatment of Endometrial Pathology in Women Receiving Exogenous Oestrogen: the Menopause and Postmenopause.* MTP Press. Lancaster.

Urlich LG, Barlow DH, Sturdee DW *et al.* (1997). Quality of life and patient preference for sequential versus continuous combined HRT: the UK Kilofem multicentre study experience. *International Journal Gynaecol Obstet* **59,** S11–17.

Whitehead MI, Townsend PT, Pryce-Davies J *et al.* (1982). Effects of various types and dosages of progestogens on the postmenopausal endometrium. *Journal of Reproductive Medicine* **27,** 539–48.

Chapter 8

The role of bisphosphonate therapy in the management of osteoporosis

Jonathan H Tobias

Introduction

Bisphosphonates are a class of anti-resorptive drug originally developed for clinical use in hypercalcaemia of malignancy and Paget's disease of bone. Over the previous decade, the clinical role of these agents has been extended to cover osteoporosis, for which bisphosphonates are now one of the most widely prescribed type of drug. Three bisphosphonates, namely etidronate, alendronate and risedronate are currently licensed in the UK for the treatment of osteoporosis. Although initial studies with these agents focussed on the treatment of post-menopausal osteoporosis (PMO), more recently, bisphosphonates have been successfully used in other forms of osteoporosis, such as steroid induced osteoporosis (SIOP). This chapter aims to identify the key evidence which underpins use of this class of compound in the management of osteoporosis, and to discuss issues related to the clinical role of bisphosphonates which are yet to be resolved.

Mechanism of action of bisphosphonates

Bisphosphonates are chemically stable analogs of pyrophosphate (Figure 8.1). The P-C-P backbone of these drugs results in their rapid uptake and subsequent retention within the skeleton, and is the basis for the tissue selectivity of bisphosphonates' biological action on bone. Several bisphosphonates are in clinical use worldwide to treat a variety of skeletal conditions. The major differences in structure of these different compounds lies in the R2 side-arm, which influences biological potency (Figure 8.2). Once incorporated within the mineral phase of bone, bisphosphonates are subsequently ingested by osteoclasts at sites of bone resorption. Having entered the osteoclast, bisphosphonates then act to inhibit essential intra-cellular metabolic pathways, leading to a reduction in cellular activity, and suppression of bone resorption (Russell *et al.* 1999).

The bone loss which underlies osteoporosis is caused by an alteration in the balance of bone formation and resorption during the remodelling cycle, in favour of bone resorption (Tobias 1999). By suppressing osteoclast activity, bisphosphonates are thought to correct this imbalance, with the result that remodelling produces a gain, rather than loss, of bone. This beneficial effect on bone mass subsequently translates into improved skeletal structure and strength, and reduced fracture risk (Tobias 1997).

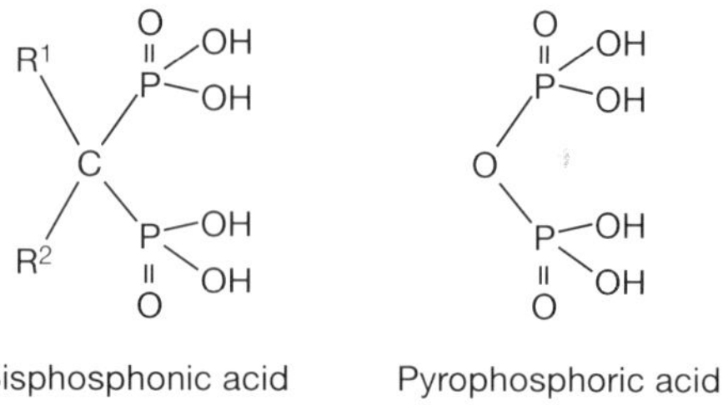

Bisphosphonic acid   Pyrophosphoric acid

Figure 8.1 Bisphosphonates are chemically stable analogs of pyrophosphuric acid

BISPHOSPHONATE	R1	R2
Etidronate	OH	CH_3
Clodronate	Cl	Cl
Pamidronate	OH	$CH_2CH_2NH_2$
Alendronate	OH	$(CH_2)_3NH_2$
Risedronate	OH	CH_2-3-pyridine
Tiludronate	H	CH_2-S-phenyl-Cl
Ilbandronate	OH	$CH_2CH_2N(CH_3)$(pentyl)

Figure 8.2 Structure of bisphosphonates in clinical use

Use of bisphosphonates in post-menopausal osteoporosis

At the beginning of the 1990s, etidronate, administered cyclically, was found in randomised control trials (RCTs) to significantly increase bone mass at the lumbar spine in patients with PMO, as assessed by measurement of bone mineral density (BMD) using dual photon absorptiometry (Storm *et al.* 1990; Watts *et al.* 1990). Cyclical etidronate was effective at preventing further bone loss at the hip, but a net gain in bone mass at this site was not observed. However, in a subsequent study of patients with PMO in which BMD was assessed using the more accurate method of dual energy x-ray absorptiometry (DXA), cyclical etidronate was found to produce a small but significant increase in hip BMD compared to baseline (Harris *et al.* 1993).

Studies have also examined whether cyclical etidronate can delay the onset of PMO, by examining whether this agent prevents bone loss in younger post-menopausal women who have yet to develop osteoporosis. Several RCTs have found that cyclical etidronate therapy can prevent bone loss at the lumbar spine and hip in this group, as assessed by DXA (Herd *et al.* 1997; Meunier *et al.* 1997; Tobias *et al.* 1997). However, in these younger subjects without osteoporosis, cyclical etidronate does not appear to produce a net increase in bone mass at either the lumbar spine or hip.

The major therapeutic benefit of treatment for osteoporossis is to reduce fracture risk. Although the study by Storm *et al.* (1990) was relatively small (66 patients in total), this provided some indication that cylical etidronate reduces vertebral fracture rate, since the latter was found to be significantly lower in the active treatment group over the treatment period from week 60 to week 150. Further evidence that cyclical etidronate reduces vertebral fracture is provided by the larger study of Watts *et al.* (1990) (429 patients), in which cyclical etidronate therapy was associated with a 50 per cent reduction in the number of patients who sustained a new vertebral fracture over the two year treatment period. Although these studies were unable to examine effects on non-vertebral fracture, epidemiological data suggests that treatment with cyclical etidronate is also associated with a reduced risk of hip fracture (van Staa *et al.* 1997a).

The amino-bisphosphonate alendronate has subsequently been developed for use in PMO. RCTs indicate that this agent produces relatively large increments in BMD at the lumbar spine and hip as compared with pre-treatment values. These changes have been observed in normal post-menopausal women (Hosking *et al.* 1998), in post-menopausal women with a low bone mass (Chesnut *et al.* 1995; Liberman *et al.* 1995; Cummings *et al.* 1998; Pols *et al.* 1999), and in post-menopausal women with previous vertebral fractures (Black *et al.* 1997) (FIT study). RCTs also demonstrate that alendronate reduces the risk of vertebral, hip and wrist fractures by approximately 50 per cent (Liberman *et al.* 1995; Black *et al.* 1997; Pols *et al.* 1999). Although a vertebral fracture is generally identified by comparing vertebral body dimensions before and after treatment, the clinical relevance of these changes is unclear. However, the rate of clinical vertebral fractures, defined as acute back pain suggestive of a vertebral fracture associated with relevant radiological changes, also appears to decrease following treatment with alendronate (Black *et al.* 1997).

Recent investigations suggest that risedronate is also of therapeutic benefit in PMO. In two multi-centre RCTs in post-menopausal women with previous vertebral fractures, risedronate 5 mg daily for three years was found to significantly increase BMD at the lumbar spine and hip, and to significantly reduce vertebral fracture incidence (Harris *et al.* 1999; Reginster *et al.* 2000). This beneficial effect of risedronate on vertebral fracture rate appeared to have a relatively rapid onset, since, in both studies, a significant reduction of approximately 65 per cent was observed after treatment for only twelve months. In the study by Harris *et al.* (1999) risedronate was also found to significantly reduce the incidence of non-vertebral fractures. In a large separate RCT to evaluate the effect of risedronate on hip fractures, which has only appeared in abstract form at the time of going to press, treatment with risedronate 5 mg daily appeared to significantly reduce the risk of hip fracture in post-menopausal women with a low femoral neck BMD and at least one additional risk factor for hip fracture (Geusens *et al.* 2000).

Although large numbers of post-menopausal women may potentially benefit from treatment to prevent fractures, it is important to target therapies like bisphosphonates to those most likely to benefit, i.e., patients at highest risk of sustaining fractures. In the FIT study, women with at least one prevalent vertebral fracture had a threefold higher risk of sustaining a new vertebral fracture, compared to women without a prevalent vertebral fracture (Nevitt *et al.* 1999). Although alendronate also reduced the risk of vertebral fractures in patients without a prevalent vertebral fracture, this effect appeared to be restricted to the subgroup of women with a reduced femoral neck BMD (Cummings *et al.* 1998). Similarly, in the study by Geusens *et al.* (2000), while risedronate significantly reduced risk of hip fracture in post-menopausal women with a low femoral neck BMD, this beneficial effect did not appear to extend to women with a normal BMD. This analysis suggests that BMD and prevalent vertebral fracture are both useful in identifying post-menopausal women who are most likely to benefit from treatment with bisphosphonates.

Use of bisphosphonates in other forms of osteoporosis

Bisphosphonates may also be useful in treating patients with other forms of osteoporosis, such as SIOP. The latter is generally attributed to impaired osteoblast function, as opposed to increased osteoclast activity as in PMO. Nevertheless, by reducing osteoclastic activity, bisphosphonates lead to a reduction in bone turnover, thereby reducing bone loss caused by the remodelling balance in SIOP (Chavassieux *et al.* 2000).

Uncontrolled studies suggested that cyclical etidronate may be useful in the prevention and treatment of SIOP (Adachi *et al.* 1994; Struys *et al.* 1995). In subsequent RCTs, cyclical etidronate was found to prevent bone loss at the lumbar spine in patients commencing treatment with glucocorticoids (Adachi *et al.* 1997; Roux *et al.* 1998). However, hip bone mass, as assessed by femoral neck BMD, was not significantly different between patients treated with cyclical etidronate and placebo. Although Adachi *et al.* did find a significant difference in trochanteric BMD between these two experimental groups (Adachi *et al.* 1997), the clinical significance of an isolated increase at this site is unclear. Cyclical etidronate has also been found to increase lumbar spine BMD in patients previously established on steroid therapy for a minimum of six months, although no significant benefit was observed at the hip (Pitt *et al.* 1998).

Recent RCTs suggest that alendronate is also likely to be a useful therapeutic agent in the management of SIOP. Pooled results from two multi-centre studies demonstrated that, in patients receiving steroid therapy, treatment with alendronate for 48 weeks significantly increased BMD at the lumbar spine and hip (Saag *et al.* 1998). Further analysis of the study by Saag *et al.* (1998) suggested that alendronate increases BMD to a similar extent in patients commencing steroid therapy as compared with those previously established on treatment. In addition, alendronate was found to increase BMD in diverse groups of patients receiving steroids, including pre-menopausal women, post-menopausal women, and men.

In a recent RCT to evaluate the effect of risedronate in patients already established on steroid treatment, risedronate 5 mg daily was found to significantly increase BMD at the lumbar spine and femoral neck after twelve months, as assessed in patients receiving steroid therapy for six months or more (Reid *et al.* 2000). In an equivalent prevention study, risedronate 5 mg daily was found to prevent bone loss at the lumbar spine and femoral neck over a twelve month period in patients commencing steroid therapy (Cohen *et al.* 1999). In both these studies, trends were observed which suggested that risedronate reduces the incidence of vertebral fracture, as also reported for alendronate and cyclical etidronate (Adachi *et al.* 1997; Saag *et al.* 1998), suggesting that the tendency for bisphosphonates to increase BMD in patients receiving steroid therapy translates into an equivalent effect on fracture risk.

Since bisphosphonates appear to be effective at reducing bone loss in a wide range of groups of patients treated with steroids, strategies are required for identifying those at highest risk of fractures in whom treatment is most likely to be beneficial. Adachi *et al.* (1997) and Saag *et al.* (1998) found that vertebral fractures in steroid-treated patients were largely confined to post-menopausal women. Therefore, post-menopausal status may be a useful clinical risk factor for identifying high risk steroid-treated patients in whom bisphosphonate therapy is more likely to be beneficial.

Several observational studies suggest that cyclical etidronate also increases lumbar spine BMD in men with idiopathic and secondary osteoporosis (Francis 1998). However, to date, no RCT has addressed the effect of cyclical etidronate in this group. A recent multi-centre RCT has shown that alendronate significantly increases BMD at the lumbar spine and femoral neck in men with osteoporosis (Orwoll *et al.* 2000). This study also demonstrated a significant reduction in vertebral fracture incidence and decrease in height loss with alendronate (Orwoll *et al.* 2000).

Concern over the longterm effects of bisphosphonates on the skeleton has limited their use in rare instances of osteoporosis occurring in younger patients, such as juvenile osteoporosis and osteogenesis imperfecta. However, following the recent report that intravenous pamidronate reduces symptoms and fracture risk in young patients with osteogenesis imperfecta (Glorieux *et al.* 1998), there would appear to be a stronger case for using bisphosphonates across the full age spectrum.

Safety and tolerability of bisphosphonates

Safety and tolerability of therapies for osteoporosis are important issues, particularly in view of the relatively long duration of treatment required. As far as adverse effects on the skeleton are concerned, it is well recognised that longterm administration of etidronate, as used to treat Paget's disease, is associated with the development of focal areas of osteomalacia. However, similar changes do not appear to occur following cyclical treatment regimes used to treat osteoporosis (Adami *et al.* 1996). Newer bisphosphonates have not been found to adversely affect mineralisation, even when given continuously for prolonged periods (Chavassieux *et al.* 1997, 2000; Harris *et al.* 1999).

An important function of bone remodelling is to remove skeletal sites which have sustained micro-fractures. By suppressing this process as a consequence of inhibition of bone resorption, the use of bisphosphonates may result in accumulation of fatigue damage, leading to deterioration in the biomechanical properties of the skeleton (Mashiba *et al.* 2000). This may be a particular concern for more potent bisphosphonates such as alendronate, which has been found to reduce the frequency of activation of new remodelling sites by approximately 90 per cent, in patients with osteoporosis, as assessed by histomorphometric analysis of iliac crest bone biopsies (Chavassieux *et al.* 1997). However, evidence that bisphosphonates increase, rather than decrease, fracture risk suggests that bisphosphonates improve, rather than impair, biomechanical properties of bone.

Amino-bisphosphonates such as pamidronate and alendronate have been reported to be associated with significant gastrointestinal side effects, including oesophagitis (Adami *et al.* 1996; de Groen *et al.* 1996). The occurrence of oesophagitis after taking alendronate is associated with several factors which it may be possible to modify, such as swallowing of alendronate with little or no water, lying down during or after ingestion of the tablet, and the presence of pre-existing esophageal disorders (de Groen *et al.* 1996). Since upper gastrointestinal side-effects are relatively common in the community, it is difficult to accurately assess the risk that is attributable to bisphosphonate therapy without an equivalent control group. Interestingly, in the FIT study, discontinuation rates and the incidence of upper gastrointestinal side-effects were similar in the alendronate and placebo treatment groups (Black *et al.* 1997). However, as subjects were excluded from participating in this study if they had a past history of peptic ulcer disease or current dyspepsia, the tolerability of alendronate in the FIT study may not be representative of that in the community.

Upper gastrointestinal side effects may not be associated with all bisphosphonates. For example, in an epidemiological study, the incidence of upper gastrointestinal side effects was found to be similar in patients receiving cyclical etidronate in the community as compared with matched controls (van Staa *et al.* 1997b). However, it is possible that the improved tolerability of cyclical etidronate reflects use of a cyclical treatment regime rather than reduced gastrointestinal irritability of etidronate itself. Whether newer bisphosphonates, like risedronate, have less tendency to cause upper gastrointestinal side effects is currently unclear. Although the incidence of gastrointestinal side-effects has been found to be similar in active and placebo groups in recent RCTs with risedronate (Cohen *et al.* 1999; Harris *et al.* 1999; Reginster *et al.* 2000; Reid *et al.* 2000), the tolerability of this agent outside the setting of a research study is yet to be evaluated.

Monitoring of response to bisphosphonate therapy

Patients who have previously sustained an osteoporotic fracture will remain at relatively high risk of sustaining a further fracture after commencing bisphosphonate therapy, since these agents are unable to fully restore skeletal micro-architecture. Therefore, if a patient sustains a fracture while taking bisphosphonates, this does not necessarily imply that treatment has failed, suggesting that alternative methods of monitoring response are required. One approach to monitoring response to bisphosphonate therapy is by comparing BMD measurements before and after starting treatment. However, recent evidence suggests that change in BMD following alendronate only has a weak predictive value with respect to reduction in fracture risk (Cummings *et al.* 1999).

Other modalities of treatment demonstrate an equally poor relationship between change in BMD and fracture risk after initiation of therapy (Black *et al.* 1999).

Alternatively, it may be possible to monitor response to bisphosphonate therapy by measurement of biochemical markers of bone turnover. Bisphosphonates are known to rapidly suppress bone turnover after initiation of therapy, as assessed by measurement of biochemical markers (Harris *et al.* 1993). Furthermore, recent studies suggest that the degree of suppression of bone turnover markers after starting alendronate is able to predict the subsequent BMD response (Greenspan *et al.* 1998; Ravn *et al.* 1999). As discussed above, the relationship between change in BMD and subsequent reduction in fracture risk is currently unclear. No studies have directly examined the relationship between suppression in bone turnover following bisphosphonate therapy and reduction in fracture risk. However, the degree of suppression of bone turnover after starting raloxifene has recently been reported to be associated with subsequent reduction in fracture risk (Bjarnason *et al.* 1999), suggesting that this approach may also prove useful in monitoring the response to other anti-resorptive therapies such as bisphosphonates.

Bisphosphonate administration: unresolved issues

Although it is well established that bisphosphonates exert a clinically useful benefit in terms of reducing fracture risk, the most efficient strategy for administering these agents remains unclear. For example, since bisphosphonates are retained within the mineral phase of the skeleton for many years, these agents may exert a prolonged protective action after treatment is discontinued. Consistent with this possibility, data presented in preliminary form suggests that, unlike hormone replacement therapy (HRT), rapid bone loss does not occur for twelve months following cessation of alendronate therapy in post-menopausal women with low BMD (Greenspan *et al.* 1999). These findings suggest that some protection against fractures is afforded after bisphosphonates are discontinued, in which case an optimum duration of bisphosphonate therapy may exist, beyond which further treatment has little added benefit.

Whether bisphosphonates should be administered continuously or intermittently is also unresolved. Bisphosphonates may be equally effective when given intermittently, in view of their prolonged skeletal half-life. Evidence that cyclical etidronate is effective in treating patients with osteoporosis (see above) supports this suggestion that bisphosphonates can be given intermittently without compromising efficacy. One of the potential advantages of this approach is improved oral tolerability, which may also result in greater patient adherence. It seems likely that intermittent oral dosage regimes will also be developed for other bisphosphonates used in the management of osteoporosis. For example, in a recent multi-centre RCT, alendronate was observed to have a similar therapeutic effect in terms of BMD when given as 70 mg once weekly compared to the standard regime of 10 mg daily, while gastrointestinal tolerability was suggested to be improved (Schnitzer *et al.* 2000).

Although the great majority of published studies of bisphosphonates in osteoporosis have examined the effect of oral formulations, intermittent intravenous pamidronate has also been shown to be effective at increasing bone mass (Reid *et al.* 1988). Since absorption of orally administered bisphosphonates is relatively poor, intravenous bisphosphonates generally produce higher drug levels, and may be more effective at reducing fracture risk in osteoporosis. Intravenous bisphosphonates may also offer other advantages over oral therapy, such as improved tolerability and patient adherence. Therefore, although intravenous bisphosphonates are currently used only rarely to treat osteoporosis, the feasibility of extending this role more widely is currently under evaluation (Dobnig *et al.* 1999).

Several RCTs have been performed to determine whether combining bisphosphonates with HRT is more effective than treatment with a single agent. Wimalawansa (1995) reported that, in normal early post-menopausal women, combination therapy with HRT and cyclical etidronate led to a greater increase in BMD at the lumbar spine and hip as compared with treatment with either agent alone (Wimalawansa 1995). In a more recent study of patients with PMO established on HRT, addition of alendronate for one year was found to result in a significantly greater increase in BMD at the spine and trochanter, as compared with subjects remaining on HRT alone, although no significant difference was observed at the femoral neck (Lindsay *et al.* 1999). In a study by Greenspan *et al.* in post-menopausal women with low BMD, combination therapy for two years with alendronate and HRT produced a slightly greater increase in BMD at the spine and hip as compared with treatment with either agent alone. Overall, these studies suggest that combining a bisphosphonate with HRT may produce a greater increment in BMD than treatment with a single agent. However, it is unclear whether this additional benefit in terms of bone mass increase is associated with an equivalent decrease in fracture risk.

In previous RCTs with bisphosphonates, cited above, calcium and/or vitamin D were generally administered to placebo and active treatment groups. There is a considerable body of evidence which suggests that correction of underlying calcium and vitamin D insufficiency is associated with a significant reduction in fracture risk (Chapuy *et al.* 1992; Dawson-Hughes *et al.* 1997). Furthermore, in the presence of significant vitamin D deficiency, bisphosphonate therapy may aggravate sub-clinical osteomalacia by inducing secondary hyperparathyroidism. To what extent calcium and/or vitamin D should be given to all patients treated with bisphosphonates, or whether their use can be restricted to those identified as being calcium and/or vitamin D insufficient, is currently unclear.

Summary and conclusion

A large body of evidence from RCTs indicates that bisphosphonate therapy increases bone mass and reduces fractures at clinically relevant sites. The majority of these RCTs have been carried out in older patients with established PMO. However, RCTs have also been carried out in other groups, including post-menopausal women who have not yet developed osteoporosis, patients receiving glucococorticoid therapy, and men. These studies indicate that bisphosphonates are likely to be effective at treating a wide range of groups of patients at increased risk of sustaining osteoporotic fractures.

Although bisphosphonates would appear to represent an effective therapeutic option in osteoporosis, several questions remain over their use. For example, how to identify and subsequently monitor patients for bisphosphonate therapy is currently unclear, as is the optimal duration of therapy, and the need to co-prescribe these agents with calcium and vitamin D supplements. To what extent long-term patient adherence with bisphosphonate therapy will be improved by the availability of newer compounds and/or novel intermittent dosage regimes is also uncertain. Therefore, although there is a strong evidence base to support the use of bisphosphonates in the management of osteoporosis, several outstanding issues need to be resolved if the potential benefit these agents offer is to be fully exploited.

References

Adachi JD, Bensen WG, Brown J *et al.* (1997). Intermittent cyclical etidronate therapy in the prevention of corticosteroid-induced osteoporosis. *New Engl J Med* **337**, 382–387.

Adachi JD, Cranney A, Goldsmith CH *et al.* (1994). Intermittent cyclic therapy with Etidronate in the prevention of corticosteroid-induced bone loss. *J Rheumatol* **21**, 1922–1926.

Adami S & Zamberlan N (1996). Adverse effects of bisphosphonates *Drug safety* **14**, 158–170.

Bjarnason NH, Christiansen C, Sarkar S *et al.* (1999). 6 months change in biochemical markers predict 3-year response in vertebral fracture rate in postmenopausal, osteoporotic women: results from the MORE study. *J Bone and Min Res* **14**(Suppl 1), S157.

Black DM, Cummings SR, Karpf DB *et al.* (1997). Randomised trial of effect of alendronate on risk of fracture in women with existing vertebral fractures *Lancet* **348**, 1535–1541.

Black DM, Sarkar S, Mitlak B *et al.* (1999). What proportion of the effects of raloxifene on vertebral fracture risk can be directly attributed to its bone mineral density effects? *J Bone and Min Res* **14**(Suppl 1), S158.

Chapuy MC, Arlot ME, Duboeuf F *et al.* (1992). Vitamin D3 and calcium to prevent hip fractures in elderly women *N Engl J Med* **327**, 1637–1642.

Chavassieux PM, Arlot ME, Reda C *et al.* (1997). Histomorphometric assessment of the long-term effects of alendronate on bone quality and remodeling in patients with osteoporosis *J Clin Invest* **100**, 1475–1480.

Chavassieux PM, Arlot ME, Roux JP *et al.* (2000). Effects of alendronate on bone quality and remodelling in glucocorticoid-induced osteoporosis: a histomorphometric analysis of transiliac biopsies. *J Bone and Miner Res* **15**, 754–762.

Chesnut CH, McClung MR, Ensrud KE *et al.* (1995). Alendronate treatment of the post-menopausal osteoporotic woman: effect of multiple dosages on bone mass and bone remodeling. *Am J Med* **99**, 144–152.

Cohen S, Levy RM, Keller M *et al.* (1999). Risedronate therapy prevents corticosteroid-induced bone loss. *Arthritis and Rheumatism* **42**, 2309–2318.

Cummings SR, Black DM, Pearson JB *et al.* (1999). How much of the reduction in risk of vertebral fractures by alendronate is explained by increased spine BMD? *J Bone and Min Res* **14**(Suppl 1), S159.

Cummings SR, Black DM, Thompson DE *et al.* (1998). Effect of alendronate on risk of fracture in women with low bone density but without vertebral fractures. Results from the fracture intervention tiral. *JAMA* **280**, 2077–2082.

Dawson-Hughes B, Harris SS, Krall EA *et al.* (1997). Effect of calcium and vitamin D supplementation on bone density in men and women 65 years of age or older. *New Engl J Med* **337**, 670–676.

de Groen PC, Lubbe DF, Hirsh LJ *et al.* (1996). Esophagitis associated with the use of alendronate. *New Engl J Med* **335**, 1016–1021.

Dobnig H, Piswanger-Solkner C, Friedl G *et al.* (1999). "SOS-HIP" Study: design of a 3-year hip-fracture prevention trial in institutionalised high-risk patients using ibandronate, calcium and Vitamin D. *J Bone and Min Res* **14**(Suppl 1), S506.

Francis RM (1998). Cyclical etidronate in the management of osteoporosis in men. *Rev Contemp Pharmacother* **9**, 261–266.

Geusens P, Adami S, Bensen W *et al.* (2000). Risedronate reduces risk of hip fracture in elderly women with osteoporosis. *Calcif Tiss Int* **66**, S67.

Glorieux FH, Bishop NJ, Plotkin H *et al.* (1998). Cyclic administration of pamidronate in children with severe osteogenesis imperfecta. *New Engl J Med* **339**, 947–952.

Greenspan SL, Bell N, Bone H *et al.* (1999). Differential effects of alendronate and estrogen on the rate of bone loss after discontinuation of treatment. *J Bone and Min Res* **14**(Suppl 1), S158.

Greenspan SL, Parkers RA, Ferguson L *et al.* (1998). Early changes in biochemical markers of bone turnover predict the long-term response to alendronate therapy in reprentative elderly women: a randomised clinical trial. *J Bone and Min Res* **13**, 1431–1438.

Harris ST, Gertz BJ, Genant HK *et al.* (1993). The effect of short term treatment with Alendronate on vertebral density and biochemical markers of bone remodeling in early postmenopausal women. *J Clin Endocrinol Metabol* **76**, 1399–1406.

Harris ST, Watts NB, Genant HK *et al.* (1999). Effects of risedronate treatment on vertebral and nonvertebral fractures in women with postmenopausal osteoporosis. *JAMA* **282**, 1344–1352.

Harris ST, Watts NB, Jackson RD *et al.* (1993). Four-year study of intermittent cyclic etidronate treatment of postmenopausal osteoporosis: three years of blinded therapy followed by one year of open therapy. *Am J Med* **95**, 557–567.

Herd RJ, Balena R, Blake GM *et al.* (1997). Prevention of early postmenopausal bone loss by cyclical etidronate: a 2-year double-blind placebo-controlled study. *Am J Med* **103**, 92–99.

Hosking D, Chilvers CED, Christiansen C *et al.* (1998). Prevention of bone loss with alendronate in postmenopausal women under 60 years of age. *New Engl J Med* **338**, 485–492.

Liberman UA, Weiss SR, Broll J *et al.* (1995). Effect of oral alendronate on bone mineral density and the incidence of fractures in postmenopausal osteoporosis. *N Engl J Med* **333**, 1437–1443.

Lindsay R, Cosman F, Lobo RA *et al.* (1999). Addition of alendronate to ongoing hormone replacement therapy in the treatment of osteoporosis: a randomised, controlled clinical trial. *J Clin Endocrinol Metab* **84**, 3076–3081.

Mashiba T, Hirano T, Turner CH *et al.* (2000). Suppressed bone turnover by bisphosphonates increases microdamage accumulation and reduces some biomechanical properties in dog rib. *J Bone and Miner Res* **15**, 613–620.

Meunier P J, Confavreux E, Tupinon I *et al.* (1997). Prevention of early postmenopausal bone loss with cyclical etidronate therapy. *J Clin Endocrinol Metab* **82**, 2784–2791.

Nevitt MC, Ross PD, Palermo L *et al.* (1999). Association of prevalent vertebral fractures, bone density, and alendronate treatment with incident vertebral fractures: effect of number and spinal location of fractures. *Bone* **25**, 613–619.

Orwoll E, Ettinger M, Weiss S *et al.* (2000). Alendronate for the treatment of osteoporosis in men. *New England Journal of Medicine* **343**, 604–610.

Pitt P, Li F, Todd P *et al.* (1998). A double blind placebo controlled study to determine the effects of intermittent cyclical etidronate on bone mineral density in patients on long term oral corticosteroid treatment. *Thorax* **53**, 351–356.

Pols HAP, Felsenberg D, Hanley DA *et al.* (1999). Multinational, placebo-controlled, randomized trial of the effects of alendronate on bone density and fracture risk in postmenopausal women with low bone mass: results of the FOSIT study. *Osteoporosis International* **9**, 461–468.

Ravn P, Clemmesen B, Christiansen C (1999). Biochemical markers can predict the response in bone mass during alendronate treatment in early postmenopausal women. *Bone* **24**, 237–244.

Reginster J-Y, Minne HW, Sorensen OH *et al.* (2000). Randomized trial of the effects of risedronate on vertebral fractures in women with established postmenopausal osteoporosis. *Osteoporosis Int* **11**, 83–91.

Reid DM, Hughes RA, Laan RFJM *et al.* (2000). Efficacy and safety of daily risedronate in the treatment of corticosteroid-induced osteoporosis in men and women: a randomised trial. *J Bone and Miner Res* **15**, 1006–1013.

Reid IR, King AR, Alexander CJ *et al.* (1988). Prevention of steroid-induced osteoporosis with (3-amino-1-hydroxypropylidene)-1,1-bisphosphonate (APD). *Lancet* **i**, 143–146.

Roux C, Oriente P, Laan R *et al.* (1998). Randomised trial of the effect of cyclical etidronate in the prevention of corticosteroid-induced bone loss. *J Clin Endocrinol Metab* **83**, 1128–1133.

Russell RGG, Rogers MJ, Frith JC *et al.* (1999). The pharmacology of bisphosphonates and new insights into their mechanisms of action. *J Bone and Min Res* **14**(Suppl 2), 53–65.

Saag KG, Emkey R, Schnitzer TJ *et al.* (1998). Alendronate for the prevention and treatment of glucocorticoid-induced osteoporosis. *New Engl J Med* **339**, 292–299.

Schnitzer T, Bone HG, Crepaldi G *et al.* (2000). Therapeutic equivalence of alendronate 70 mg once-weekly and alendronate 10 mg daily in the treatment of osteoporosis. *Aging Clin Exp Res* **12**, 1–12.

Storm T, Thamsborg G, Steiniche T *et al.* (1990). Effect of intermittent cyclical etidronate therapy on bone mass and fracture rate in women with postmenopausal osteoporosis. *N Engl J Med* **322**, 1265–71.

Struys A, Snelder AA, Mulder H (1995). Cyclical etidronate reverses bone loss of the spine and proximal femur in patients with established corticosteroid-induced osteoporosis. *Am J Med* **99**, 235–242.

Tobias JH (1997). How do bisphosphonates prevent fractures? *Ann Rheum Dis* **56**, 510–511.

Tobias JH (1999). Bone Biology and the Management of Osteoporosis *Rheumatology in Europe* **28**, 93–98.

Tobias JH, Dalzell N, Pazianis M *et al.* (1997). Cyclical etidronate prevents spinal bone loss in early postmenopausal women *Brit J Rheumatol* **36**, 612 613.

van Staa T, Abenhaim L, Cooper C (1997a). Use of cyclical etidronate and prevention of non-vertebral fractures. *Brit J Rheumatol* **37,** 87–94.

van Staa T, Abenheim L, Cooper C (1997b). Upper gastrointestinal adverse events with cyclical etidronate. *Am J Med* **103,** 462–467.

Watts N, Harris S, Genant H *et al.* (1990). Intermittent cyclical etidronate treatment of postmenopausal osteoporosis. *N Engl J Med* **323,** 73–79.

Wimalawansa SJ (1995). Combined therapy with estrogen and etidronate has an additive effect on bone mineral density in the hip and vertebrae: four-year randomized study. *Am J Med* **99,** 36–42.

PART 4

Economics, individual patient care and evidence-based clinical practice guidelines

Chapter 9

The economics of fracture prevention

David J Torgerson, Cynthia P Iglesias and David M Reid

Introduction

Osteoporosis, as well as being a serious cause of mortality and morbidity, is associated with large financial costs. It has been estimated, for instance, that a hip fracture costs about £12,000 in the 12 months after fracture with a cost to the total UK population being estimated at approximately £940 million (Dolan & Torgerson 1998).

Currently, few people at risk of an osteoporotic fracture are treated. A case control study that looked at the medical records of women aged 50 years and over who had sustained either a hip, Colles or clinical vertebral fracture revealed that only women who had sustained a vertebral fracture were prescribed anti-fracture treatments significantly more than aged matched controls. However, even among these women 60 per cent were not prescribed any pharmaceutical treatments at all (Torgerson & Dolan 1998). Not treating people at high risk of fracture is likely to be inefficient. Significant health benefits could be obtained at either no cost, that is the cost of prevention is more than balanced by financial savings by avoiding treatment, or at a modest cost.

There are an increasing number of treatments available for fracture prevention; however, to date none of the randomised trials of these treatments have included an economic evaluation. Therefore, published economic evaluations of anti-fracture treatments have to rely on economic models (Torgerson & Reid 1997). Ideally, some economic data on costs and consequences should be collected during randomised trials as, clearly, costs can be as susceptible to various biases as outcome data, a problem randomisation largely overcomes. In this chapter we will consider some of the economic issues with respect to fracture prevention.

Economic evaluation techniques

An economic evaluation has been defined as 'the comparative analysis of alternative courses of action in terms of both their cost and consequences' (Drummond *et al.* 1997). Four different types of economic evaluation are generally used: cost minimisation analysis, cost effectiveness analysis, cost utility analysis and cost benefit analysis. Measurement of cost alone, such as used in cost of illness studies, is not considered to be an economic evaluation.

Cost-minimisation analysis is generally used when the alternatives being compared produce equivalent health outcomes and therefore their difference in effectiveness can be measured only in terms of cost. Conversely when health technologies with different effects are compared , but the consequences of each can be measured in the same natural units such as life-year gained, cases detected, disability days saved, blood pressure reduction etc., a cost-effectiveness analysis could be performed.

When individual preferences regarding the health care technologies being studied are a relevant aspect of the analysis, cost-utility analysis allows the inclusion of changes in the individual's utility in the measurement of health care consequences. Some of the must commonly used units of measurement in this kind of analysis are quality adjusted life years (QALY) and healthy years equivalent (HYE). This method of evaluation is the most widely used in the field of osteoporosis therapies (Torgerson & Reid 1997).

Finally, when both cost and consequences of the alternative health technologies can be measured in commensurable units, a cost benefit analysis of the programmes can be performed. Cost benefit analysis (CBA) allows the comparison of programmes from different disciplines, i.e., health care technologies, fiscal programmes, political programmes and so on. As a result of the difficulties of measuring health benefits in monetary units, CBA is rarely used in health care; however, there is one example in the literature evaluating hormone replacement therapy (HRT) for the treatment of menopausal symptoms (Zethraeus 1998).

Lack of information represents one of the main burdens for the performance of any economic evaluation study. This is particularly true in the field of fracture prevention as, to date, there is no published evaluation using empirical data from randomised studies. In this context, modelling techniques have proved to be of great value: by making use of statistical and mathematical tools, the behaviour of unknown relevant variables can be explored. However, it is important to keep in mind that, rather than prediction or extrapolation of data, the main value of modelling is to facilitate the identification of key variables within a study, as well as to highlight the need for further research. Therefore, in future fracture prevention trials there is an urgent need to collect resource use data as well as the clinical consequence of treatment.

Cost analysis of osteoporosis

An analysis of osteoporosis costs can be useful when evaluating different anti-fracture treatments, since the costs of prevention can be partly offset with savings accruing due to fracture prevention. There have been two estimates of the costs of hip fracture in the UK. These studies, undertaken in Aberdeen (French *et al.* 1995) and Peterborough (Hollingworth *et al.* 1993), reported similar estimates for hip fracture treatment of around £5,000. However, they did not fully take into account the non-acute treatment costs, such as the increased use of residential or sheltered care, caused by hip fracture. Including these other associated costs approximately doubles the cost of a hip fracture to about £12,000 (Dolan & Torgerson 1998). Taking estimates of fracture costs and multiplying them by the estimate incidence of fractures, Dolan & Torgerson (1998) concluded that the burden of osteoporosis could be approximately £940 million. However, these total costs are very dependent upon the epidemiological source of fracture incidence (Donaldson *et al.* 1990). More recent epidemiological data have become available (Johansen *et al.* 1997).

However, these total costs are very dependent upon the epidemiological source of fracture incidence (Donaldson *et al.* 1990). More recent epidemiological data have become available (Johansen *et al.* 1997)[1]. If these data are used then the total cost estimate increases. Moreover, Dolan and Torgerson (1998) only considered the first year of costs. Uprating these costs and including nursing home and residential costs for a second year produces an estimate of £13,000 for the first year of hip fracture and £7,000 for the subsequent year after fracture. Thus, Johansen *et al.* (1997) estimated that there were 2.28 hip fractures, among women, annually per 1,000 of the population, whilst for men the corresponding figure is 0.61 per 1,000. For a UK population of 59 million (with 30 million women and 29 million men) we would expect there to be 68,640 female hip fractures and 17,768 male hip fractures annually. Combining these estimates of hip fracture incidence with the increased cost estimates give a total cost of £1,728,160,000 for hip fractures annually (i.e., 68,640 × £20,000 + 17,768 × £20,000).

Although the costs of osteoporosis are high, of more importance economically is what proportion of fractures are preventable and at what cost. In this chapter we will consider the available treatment options under two categories: hormonal and non hormonal therapies.

Hormonal treatments

Hormone replacement therapy

Hormone replacement therapy (HRT) is mainly used for the treatment of menopausal symptoms. For this use there is little doubt that it is a relatively cost effective therapy. Daly and colleagues (1993) have shown that HRT produces a modest cost per QALY. Furthermore, Zethraeus (1998) asked women with severe menopausal symptoms to put a monetary value on the benefit of HRT. He found that after treatment women were prepared to pay, on average, about £3,000 annually for the benefit of menopausal symptom relief (about 12 per cent of their income). Given that this amount is far greater than the annual cost of HRT then treatment is clearly cost beneficial.

As well as these studies looking at the use of HRT for menopausal symptom relief, there have been more than 15 economic evaluations of HRT, all modelling studies, looking at its potential for the prevention of chronic diseases such as osteoporosis and cardiovascular disease (Torgerson & Reid 1997). Although these evaluations are from a number of different countries such as Australia (Cheung & Wren 1992; Geelhoed *et al.* 1994), the UK (Daly *et al.* 1994) and the USA (Weinstein

---

[1] We are grateful to Dr Johansen and Dr Stone for bringing to our attention their fracture incidence estimates.

1980, 1990; Weinstein & Schiff 1983; Tosteson *et al.* 1990), they all tend to use very similar assumptions. These assumptions are that five to ten years of HRT reduces hip fractures by 50 per cent, and cardiovascular disease by 30–50 per cent and that it only has a modest effect on breast cancer risk after five years of treatment. However, recent observational data has challenged many of these assumptions. First, it now seems likely that the effect of HRT on fractures lasts only as long as it is taken and that once women have ceased treatment their risk of fracture soon returns to normal (Cauley *et al.* 1995; Michaelsson *et al.* 1998). Secondly, the effect of HRT on cardiovascular disease is probably less than that seen in observational data. Indeed, the available evidence from randomised trials shows no beneficial effect of HRT on symptomatic cardiovascular disease. Hence, a meta-analysis of small trials of HRT showed an increase in cardiovascular events with an average 12–24 months follow-up (Hemminki & McPherson 1997). This initial increase in cardiovascular events in the first 24 months of therapy was also noted in the only large randomised trial of HRT for secondary prevention of cardiovascular disease, although there was reduction in cardiovascular events in the latter 24 months. However, this resulted in an overall null effect on cardiovascular disease (Hulley *et al.* 1998). It is likely, therefore, that observational data do overestimate the effectiveness of HRT on cardiovascular disease (Barrett-Connor 1998).

On the other hand, the secondary prevention trial by Hulley and colleagues (1998) did note that the HRT group had a 30 per cent increased incidence in breast cancer (not statistically significant) compared with the placebo group after four years of treatment. Hence, randomised evidence, thus far, supports observational data in terms of HRT's association with increased breast cancer risk but not its ability to reduce cardiovascular disease.

Although the randomised evidence of HRT is still insufficient to completely conclude that HRT does not have a role in preventing cardiovascular disease, it has increased the level of uncertainty with respect to its cost effectiveness of treating women who do not have menopausal symptoms. However, there is evidence from a randomised trial that HRT is effective at preventing perimenopausal fractures (Komulainen *et al.* 1998). Hence, a study undertaken among women aged about 55 years showed that five years of HRT reduced subsequent perimenopausal fractures by 53 per cent. Given the low cost of most HRT preparations even if the hormone had no effect on cardiovascular events (which are uncommon anyway among women under 60 years of age) then it might still be a cost effective treatment for preventing fractures among high risk women.

There are a number of fracture risk factors which can be used to target HRT to high risk perimenopausal women. Two large prospective cohort studies undertaken in Finland and Scotland have both identified an early menopause, previous fracture history and low bone mineral density (BMD) as being important risk factors for perimenopausal fracture (Kroger *et al.* 1995; Torgerson *et al.* 1996).

In the original epidemiological papers the fracture risk is presented as either odds ratios or relative risks (Kroger *et al.* 1995; Torgerson *et al.* 1996). Unfortunately, this method of presenting risk data can be difficult to interpret. What is needed is a risk estimate which a clinician can use to estimate an individual patient's risk given the presence or absence of a fracture risk factor.

In Table 9.1, only three risk factors are considered: early menopause before the age of 50 years, one prior fracture and two or more prior fractures. We also show the effect of adding a BMD measurement to the fracture risk estimate. Using the table, a simple but crude cost per averted fracture can be estimated by taking the cost of an HRT preparation and dividing this by the estimated fracture reduction. Thus, let us assume that a woman presents with her second fracture at aged 57 and has had an early menopause. Assuming the proposed treatment cost is £45 per year and this reduces subsequent fractures by 50 per cent then her probability of sustaining a fracture will fall from 9.42 per cent to 4.71 per cent which will result in a cost per averted fracture of £955 (i.e., £45/0.0471).

Table 9.1 Population relative risk of fracture by numbers of risk factor

Women aged 50 to 60			*Annual absolute fracture risk for women aged:*	
Risk factors	*Prevalence of factor (%)*	*Relative risk if have factor versus average risk*	*50–54 (%)*	*55–59 (%)*
No risk factors	58.32	0.52	0.67	0.83
One Risk Factor	32.8	1.20	1.55	1.92
Two Risk Factors	7.6	2.72	3.51	4.34
Three Risk Factors	1.4	5.89	7.60	9.42
After bone densitometry				
One Risk Factor BMD > mean	14.3	0.64	0.83	1.02
One Risk Factor BMD in 2nd $\frac{1}{4}$	8.5	1.13	1.46	1.81
Two Risk Factors BMD > mean	2.9	1.35	1.74	2.78
One Risk Factor BMD in lowest $\frac{1}{4}$	10.1	1.98	2.55	3.17
Two Risk Factors BMD in 2nd lowest $\frac{1}{4}$	2.0	2.36	3.04	3.78
Three Risk Factors BMD above mean	0.4	2.81	3.62	4.50
Two Risk Factors BMD in lowest $\frac{1}{4}$	2.6	4.04	5.21	6.46
Three Risk Factors BMD in 2nd lowest $\frac{1}{4}$	0.1	4.78	6.17	7.65
Three Risk Factors BMD in lowest $\frac{1}{4}$	0.9	7.83	10.10	12.53

The non spine fracture incidence for Caucasian British women aged 52 is 1.29 per cent, and for women aged 57 is 1.6 per cent (Johansen *et al.* 1997). Further, the percentages only relate to the risk factors of menopause below the age of 50 years (including hysterectomy), one or two fractures prior to the age of 50 years. In Table 9.2 we have undertaken a re-analysis of risk factor from the Scottish cohort study (Torgerson *et al.* 1996)

As Table 9.1 shows, bone mineral density measurements can be used to refine estimates of risk and are probably most cost effective among women at intermediate risk (i.e., with a single risk factor). They may also improve compliance with HRT (Torgerson *et al.* 1997).

Selective oestrogen receptor modulators (SERMs)

Recently the first SERM has been licensed for treatment of osteoporosis. A promising advantage of the SERMs is that they do not seem to be associated with increases in breast cancer. Indeed, evidence from trials suggests a protective effect on the breast (Cummings *et al.* 1999). However, whilst there is trial evidence which shows that the SERM raloxifene reduces vertebral fractures among women with vertebral fractures and low BMD (Ettinger *et al.* 1999) its effect on appendicular fractures is at best only modest with a small non-significant reduction in hip and other non-vertebral fractures. Therefore, it is unlikely to be a cost effective alternative to either conventional HRT or alternative anti-fracture therapies. Furthermore, it seems likely that women at high risk of fracture (i.e., with low BMD) actually have a lower risk of breast cancer (Cauley *et al.* 1996; Zhang *et al.* 1997). Thus, the added benefit of breast cancer reduction may not add much to the benefit estimates of any cost benefit equation if women with low BMD are targeted for treatment.

Non-hormonal treatments

There are a number of non-hormonal treatments available for fracture prevention, including the bisphosphonates, calcium with vitamin D and hip protectors. As with HRT, their cost effectiveness will be enhanced if targeted among patients with the highest risk of fracture. Bone mass, whether measured by dual energy x-ray absorptiometry (DXA) or broad band ultrasound attenuation (BUA), is the best single predictor of fracture. A recent meta-analysis of all prospective studies has shown that, for every standard deviation change in bone mass, the risk of sustaining a hip fracture approximately doubles (Marshall *et al.* 1996; Hailey *et al.* 1998). However, the addition of other risk factors can improve the specificity of BMD measurements. Thus a number of studies have shown that other risk factors are important in fracture prediction as well as bone mass. The largest of these prospective studies is the Study of Osteoporotic Fractures (SOFt). This large cohort study showed that 16 risk factors (including bone mass) were independently predictive of fracture risk (Cummings *et al.* 1995). However, eliciting all 16 risk factors from patients is time consuming and a more recent analysis of the data has reduced this list of 16 down to a more manageable five: low body weight (< 58 kilos); any prior fracture since the age of 40 years; a maternal or sibling history of hip fracture; being a current smoker; and low BMD at the neck of femur (Eddy *et al.* 1998).

These risk factors differ somewhat from risk factors for fracture in younger women. Although low BMD and prior fracture are common to younger and older women (low BMD at the spine is more predictive of perimenopausal fracture than of the neck of femur (Torgerson *et al.* 1996) body weight and smoking history do not seem to be predictive of fractures in younger women. In older women, body weight in particular, possibly used in conjuction with fracture history, is useful for assigning risk. Table 9.2 summarises some recent prospective studies undertaken in older men and women showing the relative population risk of hip and appendicular fractures by body weight. As the table shows, individuals whose body weight tends to fall in the lowest quarter of a normal range (about 58 kilos or 9 stones) have approximately double the risk of fracture compared with the average.

Table 9.2 Body weight as a risk factor for fracture

Study	Population	Relative risk of fracture
Study of osteoporotic fractures (Eddy *et al.* 1998)	US Caucasian women > 65 years lowest $\frac{1}{4}$ of weight	1.9 (hips only)
Dubbo Study (Nguyen *et al.* 1993)	Australian women > 60 years lowest $\frac{1}{4}$ of weight	2.0 (all appendicular)
Amsterdam Study (Pluijm *et al.* 1999)	Dutch men and women mean age 83 years lowest $\frac{1}{2}$ of body weight	1.5 (hips only)

Targeting calcium and vitamin D among residents of nursing homes

Residents of nursing homes and other institutions tend to have a higher hip fracture rate than average. Porter *et al.* (1990), in a prospective study of ultrasound for hip fracture prediction showed that elderly women (mean age 84 years) living in residential care had a hip fracture incidence of 2.6 per cent. According to Pluijm *et al.* (1999) who looked at fracture risk factors for a similar population approximately three quarters of hip fractures will occur among women with a body weight of 67 kg or less (i.e., below the mean). Thus, out of the 26 hip fracture occurring per 1,000 women in residential care annually about 20 will be among the 500 lightest women. If these 500 women were offered annual calcium and vitamin D supplementation at a cost of £55 per woman this would cost approximately £27,500 for the 500 women. According to a randomised trial of calcium and vitamin D about 30 per cent, or six, of these 20 hip fractures will be prevented (Chapuy *et al.* 1992). Dolan and Torgerson (1998) have estimated that the costs of a hip fracture, not including residential care, amount to about £4,972 in the first 12 months after fracture. Hence, for the six prevented hip fractures there is a cost saving of £29,832 or a cost saving of £2,332 for the 500 women with low body weight (or £4.66 per treated woman). Treating the remaining 500 women is less cost effective, since the costs are the same but only about two hip fractures can be prevented, taking the savings into account it would cost about £17,556 each to prevent the remaining two hip fractures. However, this might be still considered cost effective, but this will depend upon the society's willingness to pay for such a health gain.

Targeting bisphosphonate treatment

As with calcium and vitamin D, targeting higher risk patients with bisphosphonate therapy is likely to be more cost effective than targeting lower risk individuals. Given that bisphosphonates are more expensive than calcium and vitamin D it makes sense to reserve them for higher risk patients. However, some of this extra cost will be balanced out by their increased effectiveness.

According to recent epidemiological data published by Johanssen and colleagues (1997) the hip fracture incidence is about 1.34 per cent for women aged 79 years. If a woman has three or more hip fracture risk factors then this will increase her risk of having a hip fracture by 3.35 times to about 4.5 per cent (Eddy et al. 1998). Treating 1000 such women with the most expensive bisphosphonate, alendronate, would cost £301,386. However, alendronate reduces hip fractures by 50 per cent in women with a prior vertebral fracture and low BMD (Black et al. 1996), hence about 23 hip fractures per 1,000 women would be prevented. Assuming each hip fracture, which occurs in the community costs about £20,000, then preventing 23 hip fractures will save £460,000 leaving a net treatment cost of £159,000 per 1,000 women.

Furthermore, recent evidence suggests that the efficacy of bisphosphonates is greatest among women with low BMD. Initial Phase III trials with alendronate in patients with BMD-defined osteoporosis showed a reduction in vertebral fractures of 48 per cent (Liberman et al. 1995). An almost identical figure was seen in a second trial undertaken in subjects with pre-existing vertebral fractures – the fracture arm of the Fracture Intervention Trial (FIT) (Black et al. 1996). The anti-fracture efficacy seemed to be similar to the much smaller etidronate trials (Storm et al. 1990; Watts et al. 1990; Harris et al. 1993) but the changes in spine and hip bone mass were rather greater, especially at the femoral neck. However, in the recently published second arm of the FIT trial, the effect of bisphosphonate therapy was only noticed on clinical fractures among patients with low BMD (Cummings et al. 1998). In this study, patients with low BMD who did not have vertebral fractures at baseline were randomised to alendronate or placebo and, as in the fracture arm, received 5 mg alendronate for the first two years and 10 mg thereafter, in this case for a further two years. Although broadly similar increases in BMD were noted in all subgroups regardless of the baseline values, it was only in those with BMD in the WHO osteoporosis that a reduction in clinical fractures (36 per cent) was noted. A similar enhanced efficacy among patients with low BMD has been noted in trials of the latest bisphosphonate – risedronate (Geusens et al. 2000).

Conclusion

Osteoporosis is a disease with severe quality of life and cost consequences. Available treatment options can be cost effective if carefully targeted to patients at highest risk of the disease. As a general rule of thumb the more expensive the treatment or the more serious the side effects, the more targeting of therapy is required.

Although HRT is often seen as the treatment of choice for fracture prevention there is little randomised evidence to support the view that it prevents cardiovascular disease. Indeed, there are only two relatively small trials to show a fracture benefit. However, one of these trials was undertaken among perimenopausal women and this chapter has shown that carefully targeting the treatment among the highest risk women can actually be cost saving even if there is no cardiovascular benefit.

For other treatments, there exist simple targeting strategies. As an example, we have considered using calcium and vitamin D among the frailest of elderly women living in nursing or institutional care. This strategy is likely to result in cost savings as well as health gains.

In summary, opportunities are being missed to prevent significant numbers of fractures at little cost in primary care.

References

Barrett-Connor E (1998). Hormone Replacement Therapy. *British Medical Journal* **317**, 457–61.

Black DM, Cummings SR, Karpf DB *et al.* (1996). Randomised trial of effect of alendronate on risk of fracture in women with existing vertebral fractures. *Lancet* **348**, 1535–41.

Cauley JA, Lucas FL, Kuller LH, Vogt MT, Browner WS, Cummings SR (1996). Bone mineral density and risk of breast cancer in older women. *Journal of the American Medical Association* **17**, 1404–8.

Cauley JA, Seeley DG, Ensrud K, Ettinger B, Black D, Cummings SR (1995). Estrogen replacement therapy and fractures in older women. *Annals of Internal Medicine* **122**, 9–16.

Chapuy MC, Arlott ME, Duboeuff F *et al.* (1992). Vitamin D_3 and calcium to prevent hip fractures in elderly women. *New England Journal of Medicine* **327**, 1637–42.

Cheung AP & Wren BG (1992). A cost-effectiveness analysis of hormone replacement therapy in menopause. *The Medical Journal of Australia* **156**, 312–316.

Cummings SR, Black DM, Thompson DE *et al.* (1998). Effect of alendronate on risk of fracture in women with low bone density but without fractures. *JAMA* **280**, 2077–82.

Cummings SR, Eckert S, Krueger KA *et al.* (1999). The effect of raloxifene on risk of breast cancer in postmenopausal women. Results from the MORE randomized trial. *JAMA* **281**, 2189–97.

Cummings SR, Nevitt MC, Browner WS *et al.* (1995) Risk factors for hip fracture in white women. *New England Journal of Medicine* **332**, 767–773.

Daly EVM, Barlow D, Gray A, McPherson K, Roche M (1994). Hormone Replacement Therapy in risk-benefit perspective. In: Berg GHM (ed.) *The Modern Management of the Menopause: A Perspective for the 21st Century. The Proceedings of the VII International Congress on the Menopause.* London: Parthenon Publishing Group

Daly E, Gray A, Barlow D, McPherson K, Roche M, Vessey M (1993). Measuring the impact of menopausal symptoms on quality of life. *BMJ* **307**, 836–840.

Dolan P & Torgerson DJ (1998). The costs of treating osteoporotic fractures in the United Kingdom female population. *Osteoporosis International* **8**, 611–7.

Donaldson LJ, Cook A, Thomson RG (1990). Incidence of fractures in a geographically defined population. *Journal of Epidemiology and Community Health* **44**, 241–245.

Drummond MF, O'Brien B, Stoddart GL, Torrance GW (1997). *Methods for the Economic Evaluation of Health Care Programmes. Second Edition.* Oxford: Oxford Medical Publications.

Eddy DM, Johnston CC, Cummings SR *et al.* (1998). Osteoporosis: cost-effectiveness analysis and review of the evidence for prevention, diagnosis and treatment. *Osteoporosis International* **Suppl 4.**

Ettinger B, Black DM, Mitlak BH *et al.* (1999). Reduction of Vertebral Fracture Risk in Postmenopausal Women with Osteoporosis Treated with Raloxifene. *JAMA* **282**, 637–45.

French F, Torgerson DJ, Porter R (1995). A cost analysis of hip fracture. *Age and Ageing* **24**, 185–9.

Geelhoed E, Harris A, Prince R (1994). Cost effectiveness analysis of hormone replacement therapy and lifestyle intervention for hip fracture. *Australian Journal of Public Health* **18**, 153–60.

Geusens P, Adami S, Bensen W *et al.* (2000). Risedronate reduces risk of hip fracture in elderly women with osteoporosis. *Calcified Tissue International* **66**, S27.

Hailey D, Sampietro-Colom L, Marshall D, Rico R, Granados A, Asua J (1998). The effectiveness of bone density measurements and associated treatments for prevention of fractures. *International Journal of Technology Assessment in Health Care* **14**, 237–54.

Harris ST, Watts NB, Jackson RD *et al.* (1993) Four-year study of intermittent cyclical etidronate treatment of postmenopausal osteoporosis: three years of blinded therapy followed by one year of open therapy. *Am J Medicine* **95**, 557–67.

Hemminki E & McPherson K (1997). Impact of postemenopausal hormone therapy on cardiovascular events and cancer: pooled data from clinical trials. *British Medical Journal* **315**, 149–153.

Hollingworth W, Todd C, Parker M, Roberts JA, Williams R (1993). Cost analysis of early discharge after hip fracture. *British Medical Journal* **306**, 903–6.

Hulley S, Grady D, Bush T *et al.* (1998) Randomised trial of estrogen and progestin for secondary prevention of coronary heart disease in postmenopausal women. *JAMA* **280**, 605–13.

Johansen A, Evans RJ, Stone MD, Richmond PW, Lo SV, Woodhouse KW (1997). Fracture incidence in England and Wales: a study based on the population of Cardiff. *Injury* **28**, 655–660.

Komulainen MH, Kroger H, Tuppurainen MT *et al.* (1998). HRT and Vit D in prevention of non-vertebral fractures in posmenopausal women: a 5 year randomised trial. *Maturitas* **31**, 45–54.

Kroger H, Huopio J, Honkanen R *et al.* (1995) Prediction of fracture risk using axial bone mineral density in a perimenopausal population: a prospective study. *Journal of Bone and Mineral Research* **10**, 302–306.

Liberman UA, Weiss SR, Broll J *et al.* (1995) Effect of oral alendronate on bone mineral density and the incidence of fractures in postmenopausal osteoporosis. *New England Journal of Medicine* **333**, 1437–43.

Marshall D, Johnell O, Wedel H (1996). Meta-analysis of how well measures of bone mineral density predict occurrence of osteoporotic fractures. *BMJ* **312**, 1254–59.

Michaelsson K, Baron JA, Farahmand BY, Johnell O, Magnusson C *et al.* (1998). Hormone Replacement therapy and the risk of hip fracture: population based case-control. *BMJ* **316**, 1858–63.

Nguyen T SP, Kelly PJ, Jones G *et al.* (1993). Prediction of osteoporotic fractures by postural instability and bone density. *British Medical Journal* **307**, 1111–1115.

Pluijim SMF, Graafmans WC, Bouter LM, Lips P (1999). Ultrasound measurements for the prediction of osteoporotic fractures in elderly people. *Osteoporosis International* **9**, 550–56.

Porter RW, Miller CG, Grainger D, Palmer SB (1990). Prediction of hip fracture in elderly women: a prospective study. *British Medical Journal* **301**, 638–641.

Storm T, Thamsborg G, Steinich T, Genant HK, Sorensen OH (1990). Effect of intermittent cylical etidronate therapy on bone mass and fracture rate in women with postmentopausal osteoporosis. *New England Journal of Medicine* **322**, 1265–1271.

Torgerson DJ & Dolan P (1998). Prescribing by general practitioners after an osteoporotic fracture. *Ann Rheu Dis* **57**, 378–79.

Torgerson DJ & Reid DM (1997). The economics of osteoporosis and its prevention. *PharmacoEconomics* **11**, 126–138.

Torgerson DJ, Campbell MK, Thomas RE, Reid DM (1996). Prediction of perimenopausal fractures by bone mineral density and other risk factors. *Journal of Bone and Mineral Research* **11**, 293–297.

Torgerson DJ, Thomas RE, Campbell MK, Reid DM (1997). Randomised trial of osteoporosis screening: HRT uptake and quality of life results. *Archives of Internal Medicine* **157**, 2121–2125.

Tosteson ANA, Rosenthal DI, Melton LJ, Weinstein MC (1990). Cost effectiveness of screening perimenopauseal white women for osteoporosis: bone densitometry and hormone replacement therapy. *Ann Intern Med* **113**, 594–603.

Watts NB, Harris ST, Genant HK *et al.* (1990). Intermittent cyclical etidronate treatment of postmenopausal osteoporosis. *New England Journal of Medicine* **323**, 73–79.

Weinstein MC (1980). Estrogen use in postmenopausal women – costs, risks, benefits. *N Engl J Med* **303**, 308–316.

Weinstein MC & Schiff I (1983). Cost-effectiveness of hormone replacement therapy in the menopause. *Obstetrical and Gynecological Survey* **38**, 445–455.

Weinstein MTA (1990). Cost effectiveness of hormone replacement therapy. *Annals of New York Academy of Sciences* **S92**, 162–72.

Zethraeus N (1998). Willingness to Pay for Hormone Replacement Therapy. *Health Economics* **7**, 31–38.

Zhang Y, Kiel DP, Kreger BE *et al.* (1997). Bone mass and the risk of breast cancer among postmenopausal women. *New England Journal of Medicine* **336**, 611–617.

Chapter 10

Defining best clinical practice at the level of the individual patient: tailoring management to specific age groups in men and women

Roger M Francis

Summary

Osteoporotic fractures are a major cause of excess mortality, morbidity and health and social service expenditure in men and women. The effective management of osteoporosis should therefore include measures to decrease the incidence and sequelae of fractures in both sexes. The Royal College of Physicians' Guidelines on the prevention and treatment of osteoporosis conclude that there is evidence that a number of treatments decrease the incidence of vertebral and hip fractures, but not all of these agents are equally appropriate in the individual patient.

Up to 35 per cent of women and 55 per cent of men with symptomatic vertebral fractures have an underlying cause of secondary osteoporosis, such as oral steroid therapy and endocrine disorders. These causes should be identified by careful history, physical examination and appropriate investigations, since specific treatment of conditions such as male hypogonadism, hyperthyroidism and hyperparathyroidism increases bone density, so should decrease the risk of further fracture.

The choice of treatment in the individual patient with primary osteoporosis will depend on the probable mechanisms of bone loss, evidence of efficacy in that particular situation, cost effectiveness, tolerability and patient preference. Hormone replacement therapy (HRT) and raloxifene are therefore useful in the management of osteoporotic women within 20 years of the menopause, whereas calcium and vitamin D is more appropriate in older men and women. Bisphosphonates increase bone density and decrease the incidence of fractures in post-menopausal women up to the age of 85 and preliminary data suggest they may also be effective in men with osteoporosis. In osteoporotic patients with a history of recurrent falls, the use of hip protectors may also reduce the risk of fracture.

Introduction

Osteoporosis is characterised by a reduction in the amount of bone in the skeleton, associated with skeletal fragility and an increased risk of fracture after minimal trauma. The lifetime risk of symptomatic fracture for a 50 year old Caucasian woman in the UK has been calculated to be 13 per cent for the forearm, 11 per cent for the vertebra and 14 per cent for the hip, whereas the corresponding figures for a 50 year old man are 2 per cent, 2 per cent and 3 per cent respectively (Cooper 1996). It has been estimated that 50,000 forearm fractures, 40,000 symptomatic vertebral fractures and 60,000 hip fractures occur in the UK each year, causing substantial morbidity, excess mortality and health and social service expenditure. Up to 20 per cent of all vertebral fractures and 30 per cent of hip fractures occur in men, so it is important that strategies are developed for the prevention of osteoporotic fractures in men and women (Eastell et al. 1998).

Pathogenesis of osteoporosis and fractures

There is a strong inverse relationship between bone mineral density (BMD) and fracture risk, with a two- to threefold increase in fracture incidence for each standard deviation reduction in BMD (Marshall et al. 1996). Other factors affect fracture risk independently of BMD, including bone turnover, trabecular architecture, skeletal geometry, postural instability and propensity for falling.

Bone density and therefore the risk of fracture at any age is determined by peak bone mass, the age at which bone loss begins and the rate at which it progresses. Genetic factors account for as much as 80 per cent of the variance in peak bone mass, whereas other potential determinants of bone mass at maturity include exercise, dietary calcium intake, smoking, alcohol consumption and age at puberty (Compston 1992; Scane & Francis 1993). Involutional bone loss starts between the ages of 35 and 40 in both sexes, but there is an acceleration of bone loss in the decade after the menopause in women. Overall, women lose 35–50 per cent of trabecular and 25–30 per cent of cortical bone mass with advancing age, whereas men lose 15–45 per cent and 5–15 per cent respectively. Bone loss continues into the ninth decade of life in both sexes (Jones et al. 1994), offering the prospect of decreasing fracture risk by using treatment to prevent bone loss. Bone loss may be influenced by low body weight, smoking, excess alcohol consumption, physical inactivity, impaired vitamin D production and metabolism and secondary hyperparathyroidism (Compston 1992; Scane & Francis 1993).

There are also a number of conditions which cause secondary osteoporosis. Up to 30 per cnet of women and 55 per cent of men with symptomatic vertebral crush fractures have an underlying cause of secondary osteoporosis (Baillie et al. 1992; Caplan et al. 1994), such as oral steroid therapy, hypogonadism, alcohol abuse, hyperthyroidism, skeletal metastases and multiple myeloma (Figure 10.1). Causes of secondary osteoporosis, such as oral corticosteroid therapy, anticonvulsant treatment, thyroid disease and hypogonadism have also been identified as risk factors for hip fractures (Cooper et al. 1995; Cummings et al. 1995; Jackson et al. 1989). The risk of hip fractures is also increased by conditions predisposing to falls, such as stroke disease, Parkinsonism, dementia, vertigo, alcoholism and visual impairment (Poor et al. 1995; Grisso et al. 1991).

Studies from Europe, the US and Australia show that the risk of fracture is determined not only by BMD, but also by factors associated with physical frailty and

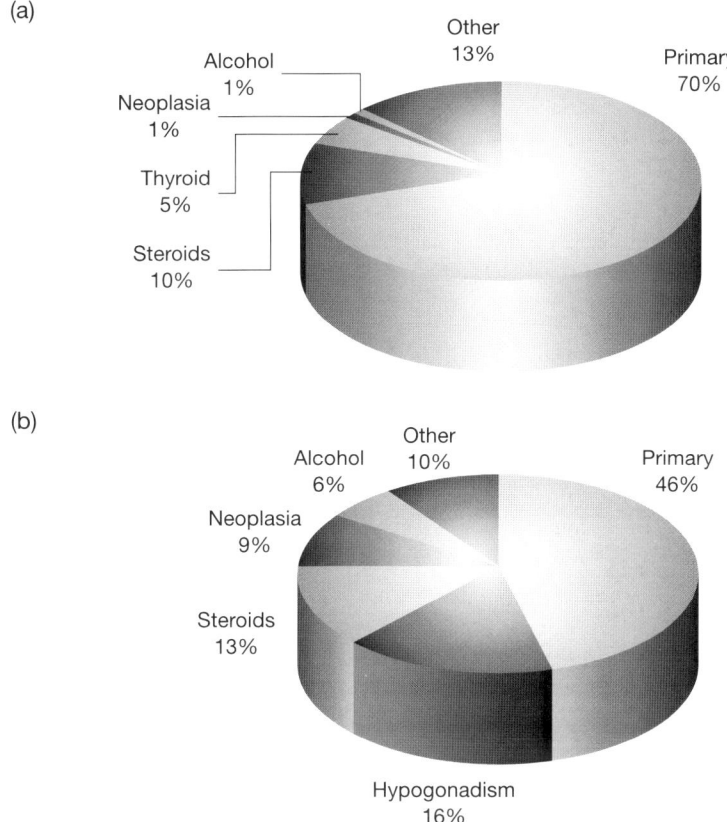

Figure 10.1 Prevalence of secondary causes of osteoporosis in women (a) and men (b) with symptomatic vertebral fractures attending the Bone Clinic in Newcastle-upon-Tyne. Data from Caplan *et al.* (1994) and Baillie *et al.* (1992).

an increased risk of falls (Dargent-Molina *et al.* 1996; Cummings *et al.* 1995; Nguyen *et al.* 1993). A prospective study from Australia showed that BMD and body sway both predicted the risk of osteoporotic fractures, but the combination of low BMD and high body sway conferred a greater risk of fracture than either alone (Nguyen *et al.* 1993). The Study of Osteoporotic Fractures in the US confirmed that bone density predicted the future risk of hip fracture, but identified a number of other important risk factors (Cummings *et al.* 1995). Women with five or more of these risk factors had at least a ninefold higher risk of fracture than those with 0–2 risk factors (Cummings *et al.* 1995).

Investigations for underlying causes of osteoporosis

As specific treatment of underlying causes of secondary osteoporosis leads to large increases in bone density, these conditions should be sought in patients with osteoporosis and/or fractures after minimal trauma by careful history, physical examination and appropriate investigation (Table 10.1). These investigations are usually normal in primary or post-menopausal osteoporosis, but unexplained anaemia or high ESR raises the possibility of malignancy, whereas macrocytosis and abnormal liver function tests suggest alcohol abuse. Hypercalcaemia indicates possible primary hyperparathyroidism, myeloma or skeletal metastases, whilst hypocalcaemia, hypophosphataemia and raised alkaline phosphatase suggest a diagnosis of osteomalacia. Serum 25 hydroxyvitamin D (25OHD) and intact parathyroid hormone (PTH) measurements may be useful in excluding vitamin D deficiency and secondary hyperparathyroididsm in patients with limited sunlight exposure, previous gastric resection, malabsorption or anticonvulsant treatment. Serum 25OHD and PTH measurements are probably unnecessary if calcium and vitamin D supplementation is planned, as the results are unlikely to influence management. Longterm studies of the treatment of patients with male hypogonadism, primary hyperparathyroidism and hyperthyroidism show increases in bone density of between 10 and 20 per cent (Behre *et al.* 1999; Silverberg *et al.* 1999; Smith *et al.* 1973), which is greater than the 5–10 per cent improvement observed with antiresorptive treatments.

Management of osteoporosis

All patients with osteoporosis and fractures should be given advice on lifestyle measures to decrease further bone loss and reduce the risks of falls. These include eating a balanced diet rich in calcium, moderating tobacco and alcohol consumption and maintaining regular physical activity and exposure to sunlight. The Royal College of Physicians, in conjunction with the Bone and Tooth Society, has recently updated (2000) their earlier guidelines on the management of osteoporosis (1999). Their recommendations are graded on the levels of evidence for each therapeutic intervention. Grade A recommendations are based on randomised controlled trials, whereas Grade B recommendations result from controlled studies without randomisation, studies with a quasi-experimental design and epidemiological studies. Grade C recommendations are based on expert committee reports or the clinical experience of recognised authorities.

Table 10.1 Suggested investigations for secondary osteoporosis in men and women with osteoporosis or fractures after minimal trauma

Full blood count
ESR
Biochemical profile
Thyroid function tests
Serum and urine electrophoresis (vertebral fractures)
Serum testosterone, sex hormone binding globulin, LH, FSH (men)
Serum oestradiol, LH, FSH (premenopausal women with amenorrhoea or irregular menses)

The effect of lifestyle measures in the prevention of osteoporosis is shown in Table 10.2. Only exercise has been shown to improve bone density in randomised controlled trials (Grade A), but there is Grade B evidence that increasing dietary calcium intake and reducing tobacco consumption has a beneficial effect on bone density and the risk of vertebral and hip fractures (Table 10.2).

As bone loss continues into old age in both men and women, specific treatment for osteoporosis should be considered in all patients with osteoporotic fractures. Unfortunately, most studies of the treatment of established osteoporosis have only recruited women up to the age of 75 or 85 years with vertebral fractures. No secondary prevention studies of the treatment of osteoporosis in older patients with vertebral and hip fractures have yet been published, but there is no evidence of an attenuated response to treatment with advancing age. Furthermore, treatment of osteoporosis is likely to be more cost-effective in older people, because of their higher fracture rate.

The updated Royal College of Physicians recommendations indicate that oestrogen, raloxifene, etidronate, alendronate, risedronate, calcitonin and calcium and vitamin D have all been shown in randomised controlled trials to have a beneficial effect on bone density.

When considering the effects of treatment on fracture incidence, oestrogen, raloxifene, etidronate, alendronate, risedronate and calcitonin all have Grade A evidence for a reduction in vertebral fractures (Table 10.3). Alendronate, risedronate and calcium and vitamin D also have a Grade A recommendation for the reduction of hip fractures, whilst the other treatments have only a Grade B recommendation for this. Although the grading of the strength of the recommendations based on study design is clearly useful, this takes no account of study size, the magnitude of the treatment effect and the patient groups studied. It is therefore important to consider these issues at this stage.

Studies of the prevention and treatment of osteoporosis

Treatments for osteoporosis may be classified into antiresorptive agents, such as hormone replacement therapy (HRT), tibolone, raloxifene, bisphosphonates, calcitonin,

Table 10.2 The effect of lifestyle measures on bone density and the incidence of vertebral and hip fractures in the prevention of osteoporosis. Grading of recommendations adapted from Royal College of Physicians Clinical Guidelines for Prevention and Treatment of Osteoporosis (1999)

	Bone density	Vertebral fractures	Hip fractures
Exercise	A	B	B
Dietary calcium	B	B	B
↓ Smoking	B	B	B
↓ Alcohol	C	C	B

vitamin D and calcium supplements, and anabolic agents like anabolic steroids, sodium fluoride and PTH (Francis 1998a). Although antiresorptive agents decrease bone resorption, the transient uncoupling of resorption and formation leads to a modest increase in bone density of 5–10 per cent, predominantly in the first year of treatment. A number of antiresorptive agents have also been shown to decrease the incidence of fractures, but this may be due as much to the reduction in bone resorption as the increase in bone density. In contrast, anabolic agents increase bone density by up to 50 per cent, but this has not been associated with a consistent reduction in fracture risk (Francis 1998a). This chapter will only therefore cover the use of antiresorptive treatments.

HRT

A number of small controlled trials (most involving less than 150 subjects) show that HRT prevents the rapid bone loss that occurs at the menopause (Royal College of Physicians 1999). Epidemiological studies suggest that HRT also decreases the risk of fracture (Weiss *et al.* 1980; Kiel *et al.* 1987). A recent five year randomised controlled trial in 464 post-menopausal women shows that HRT reduces the risk of non-vertebral fractures by 71 per cent (Komulainen *et al.* 1998). Unfortunately, the benefit of previous long term HRT on bone density decreases progressively once treatment is stopped and may be lost completely by the age of 75 years (Felson *et al.* 1993).

An alternative approach is to use HRT in older women or those with established osteoporosis, where the reduction in fracture risk may be apparent earlier. Small studies in older women with established osteoporosis (subject number 40 and 78, with mean age 65 and 68 years respectively) show that HRT increases spine bone density by about 5 per cent (Lindsay & Tohme 1990; Lufkin *et al.* 1992). One of these studies also shows a reduction in vertebral fracture incidence of 60 per cent (Lufkin *et al.* 1992).

Table 10.3 The effect of drug treatment on the incidence of vertebral, non-vertebral and hip fractures. Grading of recommendations adapted from the updated Royal College of Physicians Clinical Guidelines for Prevention and Treatment of Osteoporosis (2000). ND indicates that a beneficial effect on fracture incidence has not been demonstrated.

	Vertrebral fractures	Non-vertebral fractures	Hip fractures
Oestrogen	A	A	B
Raloxifene	A	ND	ND
Etidronate	A	B	B
Alendronate	A	A	A
Risedronate	A	A	A
Calcitonin	A	B	B
Calcium & vitamin D	ND	A	A

Tibolone

Tibolone (Livial) has weak oestrogenic, progestogenic and androgenic actions. Studies in 91 normal women who have been post-menopausal for over ten years, and in 107 osteoporotic women with a mean age of 63 years, show that tibolone increases bone density (Bjarnason *et al.* 1996; Pavlov *et al.* 1999), but there is no information on its effect on fracture incidence.

Raloxifene

Raloxifene (Evista) is a selective oestrogen receptor modulator (SERM), which has oestrogen agonist actions on the skeleton and lipid profile, but acts as an oestrogen antagonist on the breast and endometrium. In a study of 601 normal women aged between 45 and 60 years, it has been shown to prevent post-menopausal bone loss and improve the lipid profile, without stimulating the endometrium. (Delmas *et al.* 1997). In a larger study of 7,705 post-menopausal women aged 31–80 years with osteoporosis, raloxifene increased lumbar spine and femoral neck bone density by 2–3 per cent, reduced the risk of vertebral fractures by 30–50 per cent and decreased the incidence of breast cancer by 76 per cent (Ettinger *et al.* 1999; Cummings *et al.* 1999). There is no evidence as yet that raloxifene decreases the incidence of non-vertebral fractures.

Bisphosphonates

These are analogues of naturally occurring pyrophosphate, which, although poorly absorbed from the bowel, localise preferentially in bone where they bind to hydroxyapatite crystals. Bisphosphonates decrease bone resorption by reducing osteoclast recruitment and function. As bisphosphonates persist in the skeleton for many months, their duration of action is prolonged beyond the period of administration.

Intermittent cyclical etidronate therapy (Didronel PMO) has been shown to prevent bone loss from the lumbar spine and proximal femur in 152 normal women within ten years of the menopause (Herd *et al.* 1997). Two studies in women aged up to 75 years with established osteoporosis (involving 66 and 423 women respectively), show an increase in spine bone density of 5 per cent and a reduction in the incidence of further vertebral fractures of about 60 per cent with cyclical etidronate (Storm *et al.* 1990; Watts *et al.* 1990; Harris *et al.* 1993). Cyclical etidronate also increases femoral neck bone density by 2 per cent compared with the control group (Harris *et al.* 1993), but there are no interventional studies investigating the effect of treatment on hip fracture incidence. Nevertheless, retrospective analysis of the GP Research Database suggests a 44 per cent reduction in hip fractures with cyclical etidronate in women over the age of 76 years (van Staa *et al.* 1998).

Continuous alendronate (Fosamax) has been shown to prevent bone loss from the lumbar spine and femoral neck in a study of 1,174 post-menopausal women under the age of 60 years (Hosking *et al.* 1998). In a randomised controlled trial in 994 women with osteoporosis aged between 45 and 80 years, alendronate has been reported to increase bone density by up to 8.8 per cent at the lumbar spine and 5.9 per cent at the femoral neck (Liberman *et al.* 1995). This study also showed a 48 per cent reduction in the proportion of women with new vertebral fracture. Results from the Fracture Intervention Trial (FIT) in 2,027 women (aged 55–81 years) with low hip bone density and at least one vertebral fracture, show that alendronate significantly increases bone density in the forearm, spine and femoral neck and decreases the incidence of fractures at these sites by 48 per cent, 55 per cent and 51 per cent respectively (Black *et al.* 1996). In a further 4,432 women with low hip bone density but no prevalent vertebral fracture taking part in the clinical fracture arm of FIT, alendronate decreased the incidence of vertebral deformation by 44 per cent (Cummings *et al.* 1998). This second part of FIT showed no overall reduction in clinical fractures with alendronate, but there was a significant reduction in women with baseline femoral neck bone density more than 2.5 standard deviations below the young adult mean (Cummings *et al.* 1998). In another study in 359 women with osteoporosis aged between 60 and 85 years, alendronate was as well tolerated and effective in increasing bone density in women above the age of 70 years as in younger women (Bone *et al.* 1997). This suggests that there is no attenuation of the effect of alendronate with advancing age.

Risedronate (Actonel) has been shown in two large randomised controlled trials involving 2,458 and 1,226 post-menopausal women with osteoporosis to increase lumbar spine and femoral neck bone density and to decrease the incidence of vertebral and non-vertebral fractures by 41–49 per cent and 33–39 per cent respectively (Harris *et al.* 1999; Reginster *et al.* 2000). Another randomised controlled trial in 9,300 women shows that risedronate decreases the risk of hip fracture by 39 per cent in those with low bone density and by 58 per cent if vertebral fractures are present (Geusens *et al.* 2000).

Calcitonin

Calcitonin is a potent antiresorptive agent, with a rapid but short lived effect on osteoclast function. A dose response study of intranasal calcitonin (100–400 iu daily) in the treatment of 208 women (mean age 70 years) with reduced forearm bone density, showed significant increases in spine bone density of 1–3 per cent over two years, associated with a reduction in the number of vertebral fractures of 64–68 per cent (Overgaard *et al.* 1992). Another study in 60 post-menopausal women with vertebral fractures (mean age 68 years) demonstrated that cyclical IM calcitonin (100 iu daily) and oral calcium supplements (500 mg elemental calcium daily) for ten days every four weeks, decreased the incidence of vertebral fractures by 60 per cent over two years, compared with an increase of 35 per cent in a group receiving calcium alone (Rico *et al.* 1992). Preliminary results from the Prevent Recurrence Of

Osteoporotic Fractures (PROOF) study in 1,255 women with established osteoporosis show only marginal benefits on bone density with calcitonin (Chesnut *et al.* 1998). Although there was a 36 per cent reduction in new vertebral fractures with doses of 200 iu calcitonin daily, there was no significant decrease in fractures with 100 or 400 iu/day (Chesnut *et al.* 1998).

Calcium supplements

Calcium supplements were previously used alone in the treatment of osteoporosis, but this is probably no longer appropriate as more effective treatments are now available. Two studies show that calcium supplementation decreases bone loss in normal post-menopausal women (subject number 120 and 122, with mean age 56 and 58 years respectively), but is less effective than hormone replacement therapy (Prince *et al.* 1991, Reid *et al.* 1993). Calcium supplements have been reported to prevent bone loss from the femoral shaft and decrease vertebral fractures in a study of 159 elderly women (mean age 75 years) who are vitamin D replete (Chevalley *et al.* 1994). One study also shows a reduction in vertebral fracture incidence in 94 elderly women with a mean age of 75 years with prevalent fractures and a dietary calcium intake of less than 1 g daily (Recker *et al.* 1996).

Calcium and vitamin D

Calcium and vitamin D supplementation may be the most appropriate treatment for frail elderly patients with osteoporosis, as vitamin D deficiency and secondary hyperparathyroidism cause bone loss with advancing age. A French study in 3,270 women (mean age 84 years) living in nursing homes and apartment blocks for the elderly, showed that 800 iu vitamin D_3 and 1.2 g elemental calcium daily decreases PTH, increases femoral neck BMD and reduces the risk of hip fracture by 27 per cent (Chapuy *et al.* 1992, 1994). A smaller American study of 389 older men and women (mean age 70 years) living at home demonstrated that 700 iu vitamin D_3 and 500 mg elemental calcium daily had a modest beneficial effect on bone density and decreased the incidence of non-vertebral fractures by 54 per cent (Dawson-Hughes *et al.* 1997). It is unclear if the benefits of treatment seen in these studies were due to vitamin D, calcium or the combination of both. A Finnish study showed that an annual IM injection of 150,000–300,000 iu vitamin D decreases the risk of fractures in 1,186 elderly people by 25 per cent (Heikinheimo *et al.* 1992). In contrast, a Dutch study showed a small increase in hip bone density with 400 iu vitamin D_3 daily, but no effect on the incidence of hip fractures in 2,578 elderly people (Lips *et al.* 1996).

Treatment of osteoporosis in men

There are few studies examining the treatment of osteoporosis in men. Observational studies in men with idiopathic and secondary osteoporosis suggest that intermittent cyclical etidronate therapy increases bone density at the lumbar by 5–10 per cent, with smaller increases at the hip (Francis 1998b). In an uncontrolled study in 42 men with vertebral fractures followed for a median of 31 months, intermittent cyclical etidronate increased spine bone density by 3 per cent annually, whilst hip bone density showed a non-significant rise of 0.7 per cent per year (Anderson *et al.* 1997a). It would therefore appear that cyclical etidronate has comparable effects on bone density in men and women, although the effect on fracture incidence in men remains unclear. Nevertheless, a post-marketing surveillance study using the UK General Practice Research Database shows a significant reduction in the risk of vertebral fractures (relative risk 0.44; 95 per cent confidence intervals 0.20–0.97) in osteoporotic men treated with cyclical etidronate compared with untreated osteoporotic men (van Staa *et al.* 1998; Francis 1998b). A recent randomised controlled trial in 241 men with osteoporosis aged between 31 and 87 years, 36 per cent of whom were hypogonadal, shows that alendronate increases bone density at the lumbar spine by 5.3 per cent and femoral neck by 2.6 per cent compared with the control group (Orwoll *et al.* 2000).

In addition to improving bone density in men with hypogonadal osteoporosis (Behre *et al.* 1999), testosterone also appears to increase spine bone density in eugonadal men with vertebral fractures. An uncontrolled study of testosterone treatment in 21 eugonadal men with vertebral osteoporosis showed a significant increase in spine bone density of 5 per cent in six months, although no change in hip bone density was seen (Anderson *et al.* 1997b). A randomised controlled crossover study in 15 men on longterm corticosteroid treatment showed an increase in spine bone density of 5 per cent after 12 months' treatment with testosterone, whilst no change was observed during the control period of 12 months' observation (Reid *et al.* 1996). A multicentre randomised controlled trial is due to start shortly in the UK, to assess the safety and efficacy of testosterone supplementation in eugonadal men with osteoporosis. As mentioned earlier, calcium and vitamin D supplementation has been shown to reduce the incidence of non-vertebral fractures in men and women aged above 65 years (Dawson-Hughes *et al.* 1997).

Reduction of the incidence and impact of falls

All patients with a past history of fractures and recurrent falls should undergo a falls assessment. Risk factors for falling are divided into intrinsic factors, including poor vision, neurological disease and medication, and extrinsic or environmental factors, such as trailing wires, loose carpets and ill-fitting footwear. Intrinsic causes of falls should be sought by history, examination and review of medication, whereas extrinsic or environmental causes may be identified from the history and home visit. In elderly patients with unexplained falls or syncope, tilt testing may also be useful.

An important study of the prevention of falls was a randomised controlled study in 301 elderly patients above the age of 70 years, each with an apparent risk factor for falling (Tinetti *et al.* 1994). The intervention group underwent geriatric assessment, with modification of risk factors for falling, whereas the control group had the usual health care and social visits. Over the 12 month follow up period, 35 per cent of the intervention group had falls compared to 47 per cent in the control group (Tinetti *et al.* 1994). Although the difference in falls between the two groups was statistically significant, the study was too small to detect an effect on fracture incidence.

An alternative approach to fracture prevention is to decrease the impact of falls using external hip protectors, which are incorporated into specially designed underwear. A Danish study block randomised 665 elderly residents of nursing homes to receive external hip protectors or to serve as controls (Lauritzen *et al.* 1993). Over the 12 month study there was a reduction in hip fracture risk of over 50 per cent in those using the hip protectors. In the group randomised to receive hip protectors, the only patients who fractured were not using hip protectors at the time. Although this is potentially one of the most promising interventions for the prevention of hip fractures, external hip protectors are generally bulky and uncomfortable, so may be unacceptable to many older people at risk of hip fracture (Villar *et al.* 1998).

Choice of treatment in the individual patient

In considering the choice of treatment in the individual patient, a number of factors are important. These include the underlying pathogenesis of bone loss, the evidence of efficacy in any particular situation, the cost effectiveness of treatment, tolerability and patient preference. It is therefore probably inappropriate to consider HRT in the absence of oestrogen deficiency, calcium and vitamin D supplementation in women at the menopause who are likely to be vitamin D replete or alendronate in patients with dysphagia or oesophageal disease.

A number of factors may influence compliance and tolerability. Conventional HRT causes regular vaginal bleeding in 90 per cent of women. Although this may be tolerated in women close to the menopause, this is less well accepted in older women. Although continuous-combined oestrogen/progesterone preparations offer the prospect of the benefits of HRT without the need for regular bleeds, these cause some spotting in the early months of treatment, which may not be acceptable to some women. HRT is also likely to cause breast tenderness in older women, who may also be concerned about the risk of breast cancer with prolonged HRT. Raloxifene is likely to aggravate hot flushes, particularly in women close to the menopause, so may be more appropriate in older post-menopausal women. Cyclical etidronate and continuous alendronate have complex instructions for administration, which may preclude their use in unsupervised patients with cognitive impairment. Calcium and vitamin D supplements may be poorly tolerated in individuals with bowel symptoms.

The annual cost of treatment for osteoporosis varies widely, ranging from £35 for premarin to £335 for alendronate and £1032 for salmon calcitonin (Table 10.4). It is therefore inappropriate to use the more expensive treatments for the prevention of osteoporosis, unless the patient is unable to tolerate cheaper treatments such as HRT, as these are unlikely to be cost effective when the fracture incidence is low. More expensive treatments should generally be reserved for patients with a high risk of fracture, as indicated by low bone density and/or past history of osteoporotic

Table 10.4 The annual cost of drug treatment for osteoporosis. Data derived from MIMS, June 2000. Intranasal calcitonin is not available in the UK, although salmon calcitonin (Calsynar) is marketed for IM or subcutaneous use. The annual cost of Calsynar is based on the dose of 100 iu daily for ten days every four weeks, as used by Rico *et al.* (1992)

Premarin 0.625 mg	£35
Prempak C	£64
Premique	£98
Livial	£170
Evista	£258
Didronel PMO	£163
Fosamax	£301
Actonel	£284
Calsynar	£1032
Calcichew D$_3$ Forte	£69

fractures. Salmon calcitonin should probably not be used for the long-term treatment of osteoporosis, because of its high cost and uncertain fracture efficacy. The cost-effectiveness of treatments for osteoporosis is reviewed in Chapter 9.

A schematic representation of the management of osteoporosis is provided in Figure 10.2. All individuals should be advised on a good diet, regular exercise, discontinuing smoking, moderating alcohol consumption and maintaining regular exposure to sunlight. In younger women with osteoporosis, the treatment choice is HRT or other hormonal compounds such as raloxifene or tibolone. In women who are unable or unwilling to take HRT or in older patients, cyclical etidronate and continuous

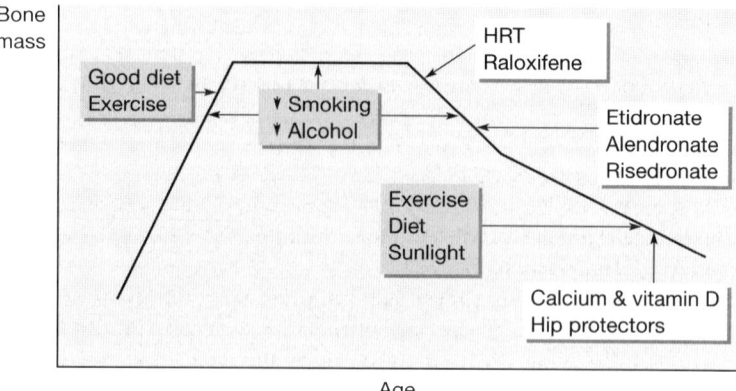

Figure 10.2 Schematic representation of the major treatment options in patients with osteoporosis of different ages, together with lifestyle measures in the shaded boxes.

alendronate are probably most appropriate. In the frail elderly, calcium and vitamin D supplementation would appear to be the treatment of choice. In patients with a past history of recurrent falls, measures should be taken to reduce the incidence of falls. Consideration should also be given to the use of external hip protectors.

References

Anderson FH, Francis RM, Bishop JC, Rawlings DA (1997a). Effect of intermittent cyclical disodium etidronate therapy on bone mineral density in men with vertebral fractures. *Age and Ageing* **26**, 359–365.

Anderson FH, Francis RM, Peaston RT, Wastell HJ (1997b). Androgen supplementation in eugonadal men with osteoporosis – effects of six months' treatment on markers of bone formation and resorption. *Journal of Bone and Mineral Research* **12**, 472–478.

Baillie SP, Davison CE, Johnson FJ, Francis RM (1992). Pathogenesis of vertebral crush fractures in men. *Age and Ageing* **21**, 139–141.

Behre HM, von Eckardstein S, Kliesch S, & Nieschlag E (1999). Long-term substitution therapy of hypogonadal men with transscrotal testosterone over 7–10 years. *Clinical Endocrinology* **50**, 629–635.

Bjarnason NH, Bjarnason K, Haarbo J, Rodenquist C, Christiansen C (1996). Tibolone: prevention of bone loss in late postmenopausal women. *Journal of Clinical Endocrinology and Metabolism* **81**, 2419–2422.

Black DM, Cummings SR, Karpf DB *et al.* (1996). Randomised trial of effect of alendronate on risk of fracture in women with existing vertebral fractures. *Lancet* **348**, 1535–1541.

Bone HG, Downs RW, Tucci JR *et al.* (1997). Dose-response relationships for alendronate treatment in osteoporotic elderly women. *Journal of Clinical Endocrinology and Metabolism* **82**, 265–274.

Caplan GA, Scane AC, Francis RM (1994). Pathogenesis of vertebral crush fractures in women. *Journal of the Royal Society of Medicine* **87**, 200–202.

Chapuy MC, Arlot ME, Delmas PD, Meunier, PJ (1994). Effect of calcium and cholecalciferol treatment for three years on hip fractures in elderly women. *British Medical Journal* **308**, 1081–1082.

Chapuy MC, Arlot ME, Duboeuf F *et al.* (1992). Vitamin D_3 and calcium to prevent hip fractures in elderly women. *New England Journal of Medicine* **327**, 1637–1642.

Chesnut C, Baylink DJ, Doyle D *et al.*(1998). Salmon-calcitonin nasal spray prevents vertebral fractures in established osteoporosis. Further interim analysis of the PROOF study. *Osteoporosis International* **8**(Suppl.3), 13.

Chevalley T, Rizzoli R, Nydegger V *et al.* (1994). Effects of calcium supplements on femoral neck bone mineral density and vertebral fracture rate in vitamin D replete elderly patients. *Osteoporosis International* **4**, 245–252.

Compston JE (1992). Risk factors for osteoporosis. *Clinical Endocrinology* **36**, 223–224.

Cooper C (1996). Epidemiology and definition of osteoporosis. In Compston JE (ed.) *Osteoporosis. New perspectives on causes, prevention and treatment.* London: Royal College of Physicians, pp.1–10.

Cooper C, Mitchell M, & Wickham C (1995). Rheumatoid Arthritis, corticosteroid therapy and the risk of hip fracture. *Annals of Rheumatic Diseases* **54**, 49–52.

Cummings SR, Black DM, Thompson DE *et al.* (1998) Effect of alendronate on risk of fracture in women with low bone density but without vertebral fractures. Results from the Fracture Intervention Trial. *Journal of the American Medical Association* **280**, 2077–2082.

Cummings SR, Eckert S, Krueger KA *et al.* (1999). The effect of raloxifene on risk of breast cancer in postmenopausal women. Results from the MORE randomized trial. *Journal of the American Medical Association* **281**, 2189–2197.

Cummings SR, Nevitt MC, Browner WS *et al.* (1995). Risk factors for hip fracture in white women. *New England Journal of Medicine* **332**, 767–773.

Dargent-Molina P, Favier F, Grandjean H *et al.* (1996). Fall-related factors and risk of hip fracture: the EPIDOS prospective study. *Lancet* **348**, 145–149.

Dawson-Hughes B, Harris SS, Krall EA, Dallal GE (1997). Effect of calcium and vitamin D supplementation on bone density in men and women 65 years of age and older. *New England Journal of Medicine* **337**, 670–676.

Delmas PD, Bjarnason NH, Mitlak BH *et al.* (1997). Effects of raloxifene on bone mineral density, serum cholesterol concentrations, and uterine endometrium in postmenopausal women. *New England Journal of Medicine* **337**, 1641–1647.

Eastell R, Boyle IT, Compston J, Cooper C *et al.* (1998). Management of male osteoporosis: Report of the UK Consensus Group. *Quarterly Journal of Medicine* **91**, 71–92.

Ettinger B, Black DM, Mitlak BH *et al.* (1999). Reduction of vertebral fracture risk in postmenopausal women with osteoporosis treated with raloxifene: results from a 3-year randomized clinical trial. Multiple Outcomes of Raloxifene Evaluation (MORE) Investigators. *Journal of the American Medical Association* **282**, 637–645.

Felson DT, Zhang Y, Hannan MT, Kiel DP, Wilson PWF, Anderson JJ (1993). The effect of postmenopausal estrogen therapy on bone density in elderly women. *New England Journal of Medicine* **329**, 1141–1146.

Francis RM (1998a). Management of established osteoporosis. *British Journal of Clinical Pharmacology* **45**, 95–99.

Francis RM (1998b). Cyclical etidronate in the management of osteoporosis in men. *Reviews in Contemporary Pharmacotherapy* **9**, 261–266.

Geusens P, Adami S, Bensen W *et al.* (2000). Risedronate reduces risk of hip fracture in elderly women with osteoporosis. *Calcified Tissue International* **66**, S67.

Grisso JA, Kelsey JL, Strom BL *et al.* (1991). Risk factors for falls as a cause of hip fracture in women. The Northeast Hip Fracture Study Group. *New England Journal of Medicine* **324**, 1326–1331.

Harris ST, Watts NB, Genant HK *et al.* (1999). Effects of risedronate treatment on vertebral and non-vertebral fractures in women with post-menopausal osteoporosis. *Journal of the American Medical Association* **282**, 1344–1352.

Harris ST, Watts NB, Jackson RD *et al.* (1993). Four-year study of intermittent cyclic etidronate treatment of postmenopausal osteoporosis: Three years of blinded therapy followed by one year of open therapy. *American Journal of Medicine* **95**, 557–567.

Heikinheimo RJ, Inkovaara JA, Harju EJ *et al.* (1992). Annual injection of Vitamin D and fractures of aged bones. *Calcified Tissue International* **51**, 105–110.

Herd RJ, Balena R, Blake GM, Ryan PJ, Fogelman I (1997). The prevention of early postmenopausal bone loss by cyclical etidronate therapy: a 2-year, double-blind, placebo-controlled study. *American Journal of Medicine* **103**, 92–99.

Hosking D, Chilvers CED, Christiansen C *et al.* (1998). Prevention of Bone Loss with Alendronate in Postmenopausal Women under 60 Years of Age. *New England Journal of Medicine* **338**, 485–492.

Jackson JA & Spiekerman AM (1989). Testosterone deficiency is common in men with hip fracture after simple falls. *Clinical Research* **37**, 131–136.

Jones G, Nguyen T, Sambrook P, Kelly PJ, Eisman JA (1994). Progressive loss of bone from the femoral neck in elderly people: longitudinal findings from the Dubbo osteoporosis epidemiological study. *British Medical Journal* **309**, 691–695.

Kiel DP, Felson DT, Anderson JJ, Wilson PWF, Moskovitz MA (1987). Hip fractures and the use of estrogen in postmenopausal women. *New England Journal of Medicine* **317**, 1169–1174.

Komulainen MH, Kroger H, Tuppurainen MT *et al.* (1998). HRT and Vitamin D in prevention of non-vertebral fractures in postmenopausal women: a 5 year randomized trial. *Maturitas* **31**, 45–54.

Lauritzen JB, Petersen MM, Lund B (1993). Effect of external hip protectors on hip fractures. *Lancet* **341**, 11–13.

Liberman UA, Weiss SR, Broll J *et al.* (1995). Effect of oral alendronate on bone mineral density and the incidence of fractures in postmenopausal osteoporosis. *New England Journal of Medicine* **333**, 1437–1443.

Lindsay R & Tohme J (1990). Estrogen treatment of patients with established postmenopausal osteoporosis. *Obstetrics and Gynecology* **76**, 1–6.

Lips P, Graafmans WC, Ooms ME, Bezemer PD, Bouter LM (1996). Vitamin D supplementation and fracture incidence in elderly persons. A randomized, placebo-controlled clinical trial. *Annals of Internal Medicine* **124**, 400–406.

Lufkin EG, Wahner HW, O'Fallon WM *et al.* (1992). Treatment of postmenopausal osteoporosis with transdermal estrogen. *Annals of Internal Medicine* **117**, 1–9.

Marshall D, Johnell O, Wedel H (1996). Meta-analysis of how well measures of bone mineral density predict occurrence of osteoporotic fractures. *British Medical Journal* **312**, 1254–1259.

Nguyen T, Sambrook P, Kelly P *et al.* (1993). Prediction of osteoporotic fractures by postural instability and bone density. *British Medical Journal* **307**, 1111–1115.

Orwoll E, Ettinger M, Weiss S *et al.* (2000). Alendronate for the treatment of osteoporosis in men. *New England Journal of Medicine* **343**, 604–610.

Overgaard K, Hansen MA, Jensen SB, Christiansen C (1992). Effect of Salcatonin given intranasally on bone mass and fracture rates in established osteoporosis: a dose-response study. *British Medical Journal* **305**, 556–561.

Pavlov PW, Ginsburg J, Kicovic PM, van der Schaaf DB, Prelevic G, Bennink HJ (1999). Double-blind, placebo-controlled study of the effects of tibolone on bone mineral density in postmenopausal women with and without previous fractures. *Gynecological Endocrinology* **13**, 230–237.

Poor G, Atkinson EJ, O'Fallon WM, Melton LJ III (1995). Predictors of hip fractures in elderly men. *Journal of Bone and Mineral Research* **10**, 1900–1907.

Prince RL, Smith M, Dick IM *et al.* (1991). Prevention of postmenopausal osteoporosis. A comparative study of exercise, calcium supplementation and hormone-replacement therapy. *New England Journal of Medicine* **325**, 1189–1195.

Recker RR, Hinders S, Davies KM *et al.* (1996). Correcting calcium nutritional deficiency prevents spine fractures in elderly women. *Journal of Bone and Mineral Research* **11**, 1961–1966.

Reginster J-Y, Minne HW, Sorenson OH *et al.* (2000). Randomized trial of the effects of risedronate on vertebral fractures in women with established postmenopausal osteoporosis. *Osteoporosis International* **11**, 83–91.

Reid IR, Ames RW, Evans MC *et al.* (1993) Effect of calcium supplementation on bone loss in postmenopausal women. *New England Journal of Medicine* **328**, 460–464.

Reid IR, Wattie DJ, Evans MC, Stapleton JP (1996). Testosterone therapy in glucocorticoid-treated men. *Archives of Internal Medicine* **156**, 1173–1177.

Rico H, Henandez ER, Revilla M, Gomez-Castresana F (1992). Salmon calcitonin reduces vertebral fracture rate in postmenopausal crush fracture syndrome. *Bone and Mineral* **16**, 131–138.

Royal College of Physicians (1999). *Osteoporosis: Clinical Guidelines for Prevention and Treatment.* London: Royal College of Physicians.

Royal College of Physicians and Bone and Tooth Society of Great Britain (2000). *Osteoporosis: Clinical Guidelines for Prevention and Treatment. Update on Pharmacological Interventions and an Algorithm for Management.* London: Royal College of Physicians.

Scane AC & Francis RM (1993). Risk factors for osteoporosis in men. *Clinical Endocrinology* **38**, 15–16.

Silverberg SJ, Shane E, Jacobs TP, Siris E, Bilezikian JP (1999). A 10-Year Prospective Study of Primary Hyperparathyroidism with or without Parathyroid Surgery. *New England Journal of Medicine* **341**, 1249–1255.

Smith DA, Fraser SA, Wilson GM (1973). Hyperthyroidism and calcium metabolism. *Clinics in Endocrinology and Metabolism* **2**, 333–354.

Storm T, Thamsborg G, Steinich T, Genant HK, Sorensen OH (1990). Effect of intermittent cyclical etidronate therapy on bone mass and fracture rate in women with postmenopausal osteoporosis. *New England Journal of Medicine* **322**, 1265–1271.

Tinetti ME, Baker DI, McAvay G *et al.* (1994). A multifactorial intervention to reduce the risk of falling among elderly people living in the community. *New England Journal of Medicine* **331**, 821–827.

Van Staa TP, Abenhaim L, Cooper C (1998). Use of cyclical etidronate and prevention of non-vertebral fractures. *British Journal of Rheumatology* **36**, 1–8.

Villar MTA, Hill P, Inskip H, Thompson P, Cooper C (1998). Will elderly rest home residents wear hip protectors? *Age and Ageing* **27**, 195–198.

Watts NB, Harris ST, Genant HK *et al.* (1990). Intermittent cyclical etidronate treatment of postmenopausal osteoporosis. *New England Journal of Medicine* **323**, 73–79.

Weiss NS, Ure CL, Ballard JH, Williams AR, Darling JR (1980). Decreased risk of fracture of the hip and lower forearm with postmenopausal use of estrogen. *New England Journal of Medicine* **303**, 1195–119.

Chapter 11

Royal College of Physicians' *Guidelines on the Prevention and Treatment of Osteoporosis*: contentious issues and gaps in the evidence landscape

David H Barlow

Introduction

This chapter has the remit of delineating and exploring areas of contention and disagreement with the recently published Royal College of Physicians (RCP) *Guidelines on the Prevention and Treatment of Osteoporosis,* and of identifying gaps in the evidence landscape relevant to the development of guidelines for practice in this clinical area.

These UK clinical guidelines should be viewed in the wider context of a progressive international development of policy in the field of osteoporosis management. An important step in this process was the 1994 Report of the World Health Organisation (WHO) working group which laid down the current definition of osteoporosis as a disease of increased bone fragility due to low bone mass and involving architectural deterioration in bone. Fracture was then defined as a consequence of the fragility (World Health Organisation 1994). The disease was defined in terms of reduced bone mass as assessed by densitometry. In parallel with this, the UK Department of Health Advisory Group on Osteoporosis had been set up in 1993 by the Health Minister, Baroness Cumberledge, and its work lead to the Advisory Group on Osteoporosis (AGO) Report in 1995 (Barlow 1995).

The AGO Report consolidated the WHO definition into UK practice and made an assessment of the current state of knowledge on osteoporosis and its management. It highlighted, as requested in its remit, the areas where there was a need for further research. Health economic analysis for the Report produced the statistic that the cost of osteoporosis to the UK health sector was £730 million per annum. The AGO Report highlighted the need for lead clinicians to be identified at the local health district level to take responsibility for developing the local osteoporosis services. This recognised that the lead clinician could originate in a number of diverse specialties involved with the disease. Having detailed many of the difficulties facing services the AGO Report recommended that the Department of Health should fund the development of National Guidelines on the Management of Osteoporosis and that a suitable base for the Guidelines would be the Royal College of Physicians. As a result the Guidelines Writing Group was set up to work on the Guideline Document.

As will be described the need for the Guidelines to be 'evidence based' became apparent in 1995 so the process of developing the document became a more extensive task than had been envisaged when the AGO recommendation was originally made. As a result, the RCP National Guidelines were published in 1999 and were able to run in parallel to the international development of policy in terms of the publication of the European Foundation for Osteoporosis (EFO) Guidelines (1998) and the National Osteoporosis Foundation (NOF) Guidelines from the USA (Eddy *et al.* 1998).

The RCP guidelines

The decision to prepare guidelines on the management of osteoporosis coincided with the introduction of evidence-based guideline methodology. This development lead to the guideline generation process being more complex than had originally been intended so that the RCP guidelines did not appear until 1999 (Royal College of Physicians 1999). On the other hand, it resulted in a more rigorous analysis of the available literature and of the gaps in the evidence base. It is expected that the resulting document should be able to serve as the basis for subsequent updates since the evidence base up to the time of analysis has been clearly identified. Updates should be able to take as a starting point the Supplement Document which systematically presents the literature database including studies presented in abstract form at major scientific meetings.

The evidence-based guideline methodology defines the processes involved in achieving guidelines which satisfy the audit criteria necessary for endorsement at the national level. The methodology defines the following structured process. There is a formal process of gathering the evidence followed by systematic review of this material. There should be emphasis on the quality of the evidence with heavy weight given to evidence origination from randomised controlled trials (RCTs) as developed in the methodology of the Cochrane Collaboration. The draft guidelines are prepared as an advanced draft by a small Writing Group and this draft is then presented to a Consensus Review Meeting. This meeting includes individuals with a wide range of expertise in the field as well as representatives of professional and lay organisations whose views should be considered. The criticisms of the Consensus Review Meeting are incorporated into a revision of the guidelines where appropriate and the final guideline can then be subjected to formal independent appraisal which determines if the guidelines justify endorsement by the NHS Executive. Following this appraisal the guidelines can be published. The final stage in the process is that the guidelines are interpreted to meet local needs by development into practical local protocols.

With the continuing acceptance of evidence-based methodology the classification of levels of evidence and the grading of recommendations in this methodology are becoming better known and are shown in Table 11.1.

Table 11.1 Levels of evidence and grades of recommendations applied in evidence based clinical guidelines (Agency for Health Care Policy and Research (AHCPR) 1992)

Levels of evidence

Ia	from meta-analysis of RCTs
Ib	from at least one RCT
IIa	from at least one well-designed controlled study without randomisation
IIb	from at least one other type of well-designed quasi-experimental study
III	from well designed non-experimental descriptive studies, eg. comparative studies, correlation studies, case control studies
IV	from expert committee reports or opinions and/or clinical experience of authorities

The grading of recommendations:

A	levels I a and I b
B	levels II a, II b and III
C	level IV

In the case of the RCP guidelines, the Writing Group involved Professor David London (Chairman), Professor David Barlow (Editor), Professor Cyrus Cooper, Professor John Kanis and Mr Malcolm Whitehead. There were also significant contributions from Dr Roger Francis (male osteoporosis), Mr Glyn Pryor (acute fracture management) and Professor Angus Wallace (acute fracture management) and the NHS Executive was represented by Dr Gwyneth Lewis. The appraisal of the RCP guidelines was carried out by the Guideline Audit Group at St George's Hospital, London, UK.

The guideline document attempts to cover all relevant aspects of the field in the text with levels of appropriate evidence graded. The sections covered by the text are shown in Table 11.2. The emphasis given to presenting the evidence base can be judged from the layout of the document. The main text extends over 80 pages with the Appendix on the non-skeletal effects of HRT involving another ten pages. The Summary and Recommendations also take up ten pages. The extensive collection of the RCT evidence base resulted in a reference list of 35 pages and the tabulations of RCTs occupies a 100-page supplement.

Table 11.2 Topics covered by the RCP guideline document

Detailed description of methodology used in the Guidelines
Background information on osteoporosis
The assessment and investigation of osteoporosis
Review of evidence on prevention
Review of evidence on treatment
Fracture management
Strategic and health economic issues
The non-skeletal effects of HRT (Appendix)
Structured account of the RCT evidence (presented as a Supplement)
Recommendations (graded)

Taking the AGO Report as its starting point, the RCP guidelines emphasise that the estimated UK health care cost has risen to £940 million per annum. The guidelines reinforce the diagnostic definitions set by WHO and reviews assessment and diagnosis, prevention and treatment strategies.

Strategic issues

In considering the approach to the prevention of osteoporosis, the evidence base was limited since there have been no RCTs comparing alternative approaches. General population intervention approaches to prevention (e.g., dietary interventions or exercise programmes) could not be supported as likely to be effective. Any justifiable intervention would have to be applied to a sub-population at higher risk of osteoporosis.

This presents us with the contentious issue of how such a higher risk subgroup might be identified for intervention. The most effective interventions are pharmacological and thus it is appropriate that there is a reasonable definition that the identified subgroup justifies the cost and monitoring of drug therapy. The best evidence indicates that simple methods based on risk-factor assessment or ultrasonic assessment of bone are inadequate for this purpose. Bone densitometry by DXA is currently accepted as the optimal method for the determination of risk but there is a range of opinion on who should be offered this investigation. Should all women be offered the investigation? This would be a population screening strategy. Should densitometry be limited to a more selected group? This is a case-finding strategy. Whilst it might seem sensible to spread the densitometry net widely in order to discover as many women as possible with reduced bone density objective assessments of this approach have suggested that population screening is not a cost-effective strategy. Ultimately since the aim is to identify a subgroup for intervention in a cost-effective manner, the focus must be on a case-finding approach employing targeted densitometry. The list of indications for densitometry, proposed in the RCP guidelines, on which to base a case-finding strategy is shown in Table 11.3. It includes specific strong risk factors and individuals in whom there is a suspicion of osteoporosis because of clinical events, such as fragility fracture, or radiological features.

Table 11.3 Indications for DXA bone densitometry in a case-finding strategy for the prevention of osteoporosis

Strong risk factors	
oestrogen deficiency	– premature menopause <45years
	– amenorrhoea >1 year
	– primary hypogonadism
	– anorexia nervosa
corticosteroid therapy (>7.5mg/day for 1 year)	
maternal history of hip fracture	
low BMI (<19)	
potential causes of secondary osteoporosis	
• malabsorption syndromes	
• primary hypoparathyroidism	
• post-transplantation	
• chronic renal failure	
• hyperthyroidism	
• prolonged immobilisation	
• Cushing's syndrome	
Radiographic osteopenia and/or vertebral deformity	
Previous fragility fracture	
Loss of height, thoracic kyphosis (after x-ray confirmation)	

Densitometry

The criteria for densitometry are consistent with other reports in the field and represent the core indication for densitometry. Other indications for densitometry are more contentious but would be appropriate if densitometry were available. These other indications are, first, in the monitoring of the response to bone active therapy, and secondly, to assist in clinical decision making where the result of the densitometry would be likely to affect clinical decision making. These latter indications would significantly increase the expected volume of densitometry scans required.

Currently the facilities for bone densitometry and the funding of scans are limited in many parts of the UK. Although the core list of indications for densitometry listed in Table 11.3 is widely accepted as appropriate, many districts lack funding to enable this list of indications to be fulfilled. In that context those districts which have difficulty funding the core list have little prospect of funding the latter two indications listed. Local circumstances and priority setting will have a major effect on the local management protocol that will result from the RCP guidelines. The situation will be further complicated in an, as yet, uncertain fashion when local funding decisions come under the jurisdiction of a multiplicity of Primary Care Groups. Will densitometry be more or less available in this new funding environment?

A recent National Osteoporosis Society survey of general practitioners has provided information on primary care access to densitometry and its use (National

Osteoporosis Society 1999). Of those who had access to densitometry assessment a majority had access via consultant referral. The analysis of which patients the general practitioners were referring for densitometry indicates that many general practitioners in the survey were applying approaches to densitometry outside the RCP guidelines (Table 11.4).

Table 11.4 Policy on the use of bone densitometry by general practitioners surveyed by the National Osteoporosis Society, 1999

Densitometry policy	GPs using policy (%)
All menopausal women	24
All women 50 +	13
All men and women 50 +	5
Anyone with low trauma fracture	82
Patients on corticosteroids	76
Early menopause	80
Family history	81

The issues surrounding the use of densitometry are, and will remain, a source of controversy. Views range from those who would wish a relatively liberal approach to densitometry at one extreme to those who are resistant to making resources for densitometry available even for the justifiable indications as presented in the RCP guidelines. It is to be hoped that the core list of indications given in Table 11.3 will be applied as a minimum standard for the identification of individuals with osteoporosis now or in a reasonable timescale.

Terminology

Another area of contention is an unavoidable issue of terminology. This relates to the use of terminology to define the focus of management. Should the terminology be centred on osteoporosis or on its major consequence, osteoporotic fracture?

The RCP guidelines have adopted the former approach, which it was judged would be consistent with approaches taken in the UK and US drug regulatory guidelines. Those guidelines state that drugs used in prevention must have been tested for effectiveness in individuals with normal bone density, and that drugs used in treatment must have been tested for efficacy in individuals with bone density in the osteoporotic range. In addition, this set of definitions is directly consistent with the focus on bone density embodied in the WHO definition of osteoporosis. In that definition, osteoporosis is defined in terms of a reduced bone mass threshold (-2.5 SD) and does not demand that fracture has already occurred by the time of the assessment. On that basis the definition centres on osteoporosis, the term 'prevention' referring to the prevention of osteoporosis and the term 'treatment' referring to interventions in individuals who have osteoporosis with the intention of preventing fracture. The alternative approach that was not adopted in the RCP guidelines is to centre the definition on fracture so that 'prevention' applies to all interventions both in those who do not yet have osteoporosis and in those who do have osteoporosis but have not yet sustained a fracture. In this definition 'treatment' only applies to the use of therapies to minimise the risk of further fracture by counteracting the progression of osteoporosis.

The author can agree with the logic of grouping together all subjects who might be using treatment in order to prevent fracture since treatments are generally effective whether or not the individual has already lost enough bone mass to be classified as having osteoporosis. On the other hand, it is sensible that the use of the terms 'prevention' and 'treatment' should be consistent with the bone density based definition of osteoporosis with prevention applying until the subject has developed osteoporosis as employed by the drug regulatory agencies. This helps keep the focus on the disease and its diagnosis. This has the advantages first of maintaining densitometry at the centre of the subject and secondly, that prevention and treatment studies will involve subjects with more consistency of bone mass in each group than with the fracture based definition. This latter point is particularly important since it determines that treatment studies will be likely to involve sufficient fractures to provide fracture end point data whereas prevention studies will involve groups which cannot be expected to provide fracture end point data. Inevitably bone densitometry will be the focus in these prevention studies.

Treatment option league tables

The evidence-based guidelines can be criticised for not being able to provide a league table of the prevention and treatment options. It is entirely understandable that clinicians wish to have a definite first choice agent for each situation. Using the evidence on efficacy it is possible to show which interventions maintain bone density and in some cases that there is a reduction in fracture rates. The Supplement to the RCP guidelines systematically presents that evidence for each of the available therapies. These randomised controlled trials show whether the intervention can achieve satisfactory end point outcomes, usually compared with no treatment or placebo. Only rarely do the trials directly compare therapies. For this reason we have no good evidence base from which to conclude that there is one particularly treatment of superior efficacy. This is particularly the case in the osteoporosis prevention context where the realistic end point is bone density change. Although there are very few studies comparing therapies in prevention, the main therapies having a similar action by reducing bone turnover as resorption inhibitors, the single agent studies provide no evidence to suggest that head-to-head studies would be likely to yield major differences in efficacy. With osteoporosis treatment studies again we lack head-to-head comparisons but at least some of the single agent studies provide outcome information on fracture end points. Thus in the treatment context it is possible to show that some of the options have demonstrated efficacy in terms of an end point, fracture, of greater direct clinical value than bone density changes. These treatment options may have a similar effect on bone density to other options but by providing fracture data it is appropriate that this evidence is given weight in choosing one therapy against other choices.

In consideration of the limitations outlined, the RCP guidelines attempt to provide a balanced comparison of the prevention and treatment options as shown in Tables 11.5 and 11.6 respectively in the format used in the RCP guideline document. Not only do the Tables show the end points to which the efficacy data relate but also they indicate if the evidence is of high quality (level A) being based on randomised controlled trials or weaker.

Table 11.5 Options and the weight of evidence for their efficacy in the prevention of osteoporosis (as presented in the RCP Guidelines)

Intervention	Bone mineral density	Vertebral fracture	Hip fracture
Exercise	A	B	B
Pharmacological calcium (+/- vit D)	A	B	B
Dietary calcium	B	B	B
Smoking cessation	B	B	B
Reduced alcohol consumption	C	C	B
Oestrogen	A	B	B
Raloxifene	A	A	—
Etidronate	A	—	—
Alendronate	A	—	—

It should be noted that, since the publication of the RCP Guidelines, the level A evidence on the effect of Raloxifene on the vertebral fracture end point was incorrectly placed in the prevention table (Table 11.5). It should have been placed in the treatment table (Table 11.6) since the subjects in that large trial had osteoporosis at entry to the study. The licence for Raloxifene at that time was for the prevention of osteoporosis so Raloxifene should have been included in Table 11.6 marked with an asterisk to indicate that there was no UK licence for the treatment of osteoporosis but showing that there is level A evidence for its action on vertebral fracture. Subsequently, a treatment licence has been granted.

Protocols and algorithms

A similar difficulty is associated with the other clinical requirement which was not provided in the RCP guidelines: the desire to have clear algorithms to guide clinical practice. The author believes that it is unfair to criticise the guidelines for omitting practical algorithms because in the defined process of evidence-based guideline

Table 11.6 Options and the weight of evidence for their efficacy in the treatment of osteoporosis (as presented in the RCP Guidelines)

Intervention	Bone mineral density	Vertebral fracture	Hip fracture
Calcium (+/- Vit D)	A	A	B
Oestrogen	A	A	B
Alendronate	A	A	A
Etidronate	A	A	B
Calcitonin	A	A	B
Fluoride *	A	A?	—
Anabolic steroids	A	—	B
Calcitriol	A	A?	C

* not currently licensed in UK for use in osteoporosis but used in specialist centres
? inconsistent data

development these are usually developed as a component of the local practice protocols which are developed locally, based on the guidance provided by the guidelines. This ensures that the therapeutic algorithm fits with local clinical circumstances. The clinical algorithms are generally concerned with strategy and it is unusual to find that such questions of strategy have been explored in randomised controlled trials. Without that evidence definitive algorithms are not feasible since, on the basis of the evidence available, different groups of experts could easily come up with different algorithms. If this is the case it is best that local experts use the evidence based recommendations of the Guidelines to design locally relevant algorithms.

These algorithms will be expected to take into consideration not only the weight of evidence for efficacy but also any risks and side-effects associated with different options, their ease of use, their relative costs and any particular issues relevant to the local circumstances. In the RCP guidelines we gave an example of a cost-effectiveness estimate for fracture prevention which is shown in Table 11.7.

Table 11.7 Estimated cost-effectiveness of preventing vertebral fractures in subjects with vertebral osteoporosis – assuming predicted 60 per cent reduction in fractures

Cost per averted fracture	
Conjugated oestrogens	- £138
Transdermal oestrogen	- £560
Cyclical etidronate	- £1,880
Intranasal calcitonin	- £25,000

Gulfs in the evidence landscape

Sadly there are many areas where evidence is lacking at present. These areas include the need for comparative evidence on alternative densitometry policies, and the need for clinical end point evidence on the use of sex hormones in the prevention of osteoporosis or in the elderly. We also have little information on the effects of the co-ordinated use of different agents at different stages in life or on the co-ordination of services for people with osteoporosis.

Conclusion

The RCP Guidelines on the Prevention and Treatment of Osteoporosis, published in 1999, present the evidence landscape on osteoporosis at the end of the twentieth century. They provide recommendations, based on the best evidence, on the provision of services in the field. The implementation of these recommendations demands action from health authorities and primary care groups who will determine spending priorities in each locality and the potential for a transfer of resources into densitometry. Any such new resources must be carefully managed because the inappropriate application of densitometry outside the suggested indications would consume resources in an ill-focused manner as a form of non-systematic population screening. Whilst appropriate use of densitometry has the potential to be a cost-effective option, an ill-managed, open-ended use of densitometry would undermine the local approach to osteoporosis and weaken the case for osteoporosis when weighed against the competing claims of emerging guidelines in other fields when spending priorities are being set.

What is now required is that the RCP guidelines are translated into local practice protocols and are endorsed by those responsible for deciding on local priorities. Those in the field must maintain pressure at the local level and national organisations, including the National Osteoporosis Society, must maintain awareness that osteoporosis is a disease which causes such suffering and health care costs that it deserves to be high on priority setting lists.

Postscript

In response to the continuing requests from many professionals in the field that there might be a management algorithm linked with the RCP Guidelines, the RCP Guidelines Writing Group collaborated with a group nominated by the Bone and Tooth Society to produce a short supplement to the RCP Guidelines document which provided an agreed unifying management algorithm. In addition the opportunity was taken of briefly updating the data on treatments to incorporate significant new data published between Autumn 1998 and Spring 2000 and not able to be included in the RCP Guidelines published in March 1999. The updated intervention table amalgamates the interventions into a single table (Table 11.8). The management algorithm is shown below (Figure 11.1). The Supplement is being incorporated with the full RCP.

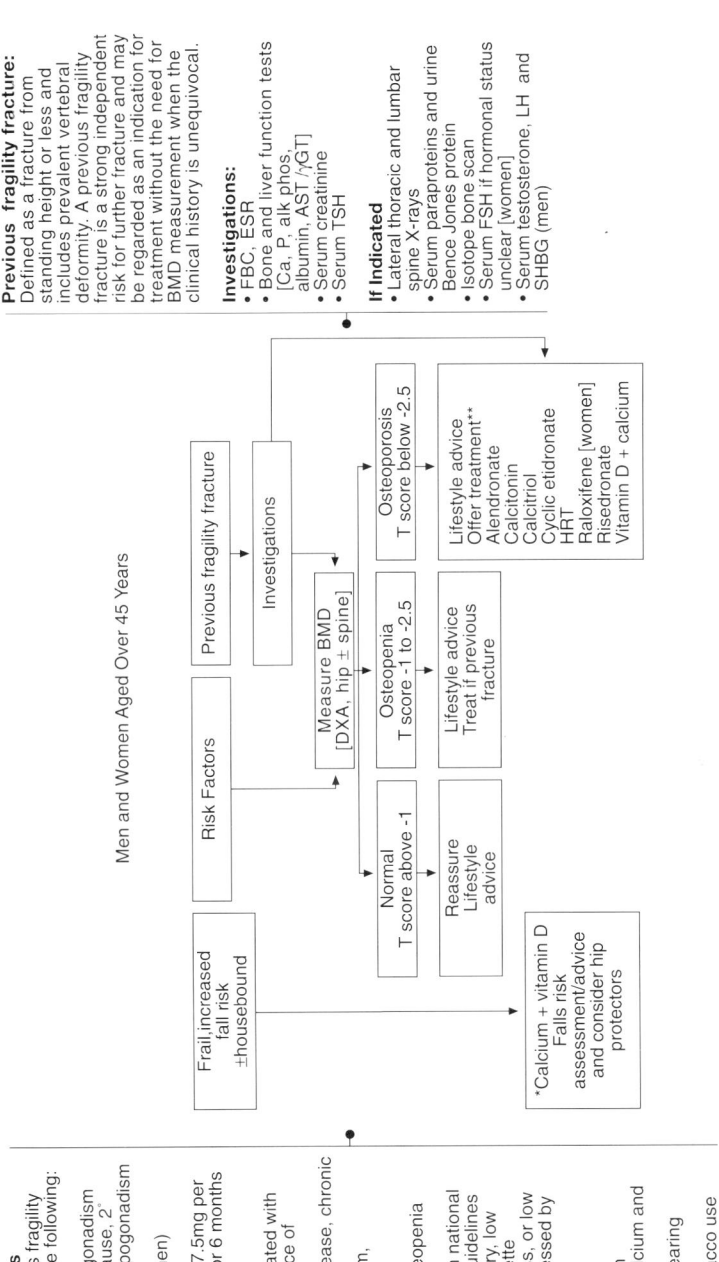

Major Risk Factors
(other than previous fragility fracture) include the following:

1. Untreated hypogonadism (premature menopause, 2° amenorrhoea, 1° hypogonadism in women; 1° or 2° hypogonadism in men)

2. Glucocorticoids [7.5mg per day prednisolone for 6 months or more]#

3. Diseases associated with increased prevalence of osteoporosis (e.g. gastrointestinal disease, chronic liver disease, hyperparathyroidism, hyperthyroidism)

4. Radiological osteopenia

Other risk factors in national and international guidelines include family history, low body weight, cigarette smoking, height loss, or low bone mass as assessed by other techniques.

Lifestyle advice:
• Adequate nutrition especially with calcium and vitamin D
• Regular weight bearing exercise
• Avoidance of tobacco use and alcohol abuse

Previous fragility fracture:
Defined as a fracture from standing height or less and includes prevalent vertebral deformity. A previous fragility fracture is a strong independent risk for further fracture and may be regarded as an indication for treatment without the need for BMD measurement when the clinical history is unequivocal.

Investigations:
• FBC, ESR
• Bone and liver function tests [Ca, P, alk phos, albumin, AST /γGT]
• Serum creatinine
• Serum TSH

If Indicated
• Lateral thoracic and lumbar spine X-rays
• Serum paraproteins and urine Bence Jones protein
• Isotope bone scan
• Serum FSH if hormonal status unclear [women]
• Serum testosterone, LH and SHBG (men)

Men and Women Aged Over 45 Years

Risk Factors — Previous fragility fracture

Frail, increased fall risk ±housebound

Investigations

Measure BMD [DXA, hip ± spine]

Normal T score above -1 → Reassure Lifestyle advice

Osteopenia T score -1 to -2.5 → Lifestyle advice Treat if previous fracture

Osteoporosis T score below -2.5 → Lifestyle advice / Offer treatment** / Alendronate / Calcitonin / Calcitriol / Cyclic etidronate / HRT / Raloxifene [women] / Risedronate / Vitamin D + calcium

*Calcium + vitamin D Falls risk assessment/advice and consider hip protectors

For men aged less than 65 years men specialist referral should be considered
*Recommended daily dose 0.5-1g and 800 IU respectively
#Refer to previously published guidelines

**Treatments listed in alphabetical order. Vitamin D and calcium are generally regarded as adjuncts to treatment.
HRT: oestrogen in women, testosterone in hypogonadal men.

Figure 11.1 Management algorithm. Reproduced, with permission, from *Guidelines on the Prevention and Treatment of Osteoporosis*, Royal College of Physicians, 2000.

Table 11.8 Anti-fracture efficacy of interventions in postmenopausal osteoporotic women: grade of recommendations. Reproduced, with permission, from *Guidelines on the Prevention and Treatment of Osteoporosis*, Royal College of Physicians, 2000.

	Spine	Non-vertebral	Hip
Alendronate	A	A	A
Calcitonin	A	B	B
Calcitriol	A	A	nd
Calcium	A	B	B
Calcium + vit D	nd	A	A
Cyclic etidronate	A	B	B
Hip protectors	–	–	A
HRT	A	A	B
Physical exercise	nd	B	B
Raloxifene	A	nd	nd
Risedronate	A	A	A
Tibolone	nd	nd	nd
Vitamin D	nd	B	B

nd: not demonstrated

Guidelines document folder which already contains the Guidelines text document and the Supplement of Randomised Controlled Trials. The new updated supplement is being distributed widely to many GPs and hospital specialists.

References

AHCPR (1992). Agency for Health Care Policy and Research.

Barlow DH (1995). *Report of the Advisory Group on Osteoporosis.* London: Department of Health.

Eddy D *et al.* (1998). *Osteoporosis: Review of the Evidence for Prevention, Diagnosis and Treatment and Cost Effectiveness Analysis. The Basis for a Guideline for the Medical Management of Osteoporosis.* USA: National Osteoporosis Foundation.

European Foundation for Osteoporosis (1998). *Guidelines for Diagnosis and Management of Osteoporosis.*

National Osteoporosis Society (1999). *General Practitioner Densitometry Survey.* Bath: National Osteoporosis Society.

Royal College of Physicians (1999). *Guidelines for the Prevention and Treatment of Osteoporosis.* London: Royal College of Physicians.

World Health Organisation (1994). *Assessment of Fracture Risk and its Application to Screening for Postmenopausal Osteoporosis.* Technical Report Series 843. Geneva: World Health Organisation.

Index